FITNESS FOR S...

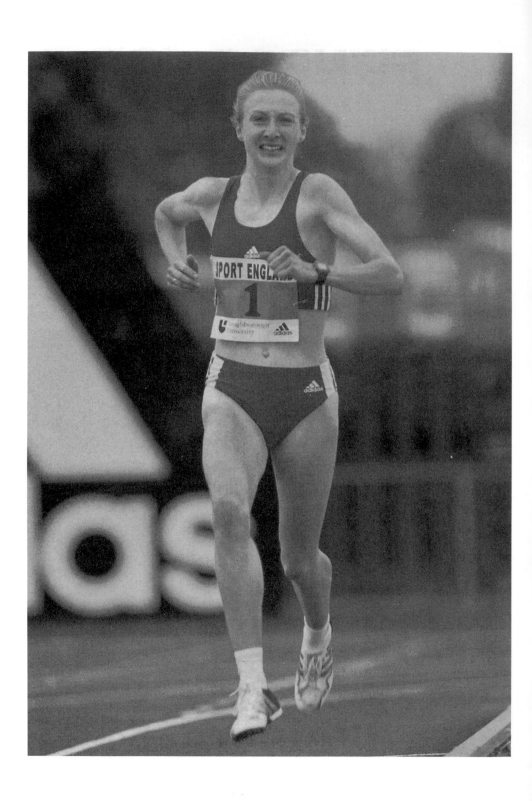

FITNESS FOR SPORT

Rex Hazeldine

The Crowood Press

First published in 1985 by
The Crowood Press Ltd
Ramsbury, Marlborough
Wiltshire SN8 2HR

Revised edition 2000

British Library Cataloguing-in-Publication Data
A catalogue for this book is available from the British Library.

ISBN 1 86126 336 8

Line illustrations by Annette Findlay.
Photo previous page: Paula Radcliffe (Ian Hebden).

Acknowledgements
Shiela Hazeldine and Dr Paul Cherry.

Photographic Acknowledgements
Photos by the Audio-Visual Services of Loughborough University, except where otherwise credited.

Dedication
To WJH

Typefaces used: Galliard and Franklin Gothic.

Typeset and designed by
D & N Publishing
Baydon, Wiltshire.

Printed and bound in Great Britain by JW Arrowsmith, Bristol.

Contents

Forewords

I welcome the publication of *Fitness for Sport* because it provides the reader with a sound background to the various methods of fitness training. Rex Hazeldine has conveyed his considerable knowledge and experience of the principles of fitness training in a clear and yet uncompromising style. At the practical level, the exercises in this book are those which have, through years of experience, been labelled 'tried, tested and found satisfactory'. Therefore I would commend this book to all those who, at whatever level, aim to improve their fitness for their sport.

Professor Clyde Williams,
Loughborough University

In our appreciation of top level sport, the high degree of skill that is shown often leads us to ignore one important and very basic ingredient – preparation.

In *Fitness for Sport*, Rex Hazeldine outlines clearly the theory behind the acquisition of fitness and details a variety of approaches to fitness training that are specific to the needs of the individual.

I am delighted to recommend this book to all those who are interested in the pursuit of fitness for its own sake, or who appreciate the need for preparation as the basis for improved performance. It is a book that will appeal at all levels of sport, will lead towards a greater understanding of fitness theory, and ultimately to more people enjoying the many diverse pleasures that sport can offer.

David Moorcroft
Chief Executive, UK Athletics

Rex Hazeldine's book is aimed at the athlete, a word defined in the Oxford Dictionary, he tells us, as 'a competitor or skilled performer, a robust or vigorous person'.

In other words, whether you are chasing gold or simply sweating away a touch of social over-indulgence, *Fitness for Sport* is intended to inform, warn, guide and encourage you. As a former professional sportsman, now reduced to irregular but, nonetheless, enthusiastic performance, I feel that Rex has succeeded in his objective. There is something for everyone, set out clearly and concisely, and backed up by excellent visual examples. We may still 'fail', but after reading this book it won't be as a result of bad 'preparation'.

Bob Wilson
Presenter, ITV Sport

Introduction

My deep interest and study into the principles of physical fitness and training began developing in earnest when devising courses for undergraduate students of physical education and sports science at Loughborough University. These courses were presented to fill a gap disclosed in the teaching of the undergraduates, and evident in my own training and development as a physical educationist. Although as a profession we study sports science, including such areas as functional anatomy and exercise physiology, together with practical activities, i.e. games, athletics, swimming and gymnastics, we have sometimes failed to develop with students of the subject an in-depth knowledge and an understanding of physical fitness and methods of training, surely a basic essential of physical education.

This development coincided with a period when society was taking more interest in exercise and health related fitness as expressed, for example, by the expansion of marathon and half-marathon events, which has brought a demand for more knowledge. So, through Summer School courses held at the University and by demands from other centres both nationally and internationally, I was encouraged to develop ideas and knowledge in all aspects of fitness to satisfy a variety of needs.

Perhaps it was fortunate that, as the rugby football 1st XV coach at Loughborough University, I had a good opportunity to put these ideas and knowledge into practice, and I am convinced that, although many factors contribute to effective performance, the fitness level of the players had considerable influence on their successes in those days. Further, this thinking has been reinforced by the results which have been obtained after working on fitness programmes recommended to and adopted by high-level performers in rugby football and other sports.

I was fortunate to be the Rugby Football Union's National Fitness Adviser and the England Rugby Team's Fitness Coach for seven years, as well as fitness adviser to the Great Britain's Women's Hockey Squad that won a bronze medal at the Barcelona Olympics in 1992. All these athletes seek training programmes which are based on sound physiological principles and which help them to reach an optimum level of fitness for their sport. I am currently Fitness Director of the Rugby Football Union for Women and direct their Sport Science Programme. The British Olympic Association appointed me as their Conditioning and Fitness Consultant to assist with establishing a Register of high-level Fitness Specialists on a national basis, in order to provide an approved and quality advisory service to top athletes in the British Isles.

Fitness for Sport is aimed not only at teachers, coaches, students and performers who would appreciate the necessity of studying physical fitness and methods of training; the book, I hope, will be of value also to any person participating in any sporting activity whether at supreme competitor level or just indulging in jogging for fun and exercise.

Incidentally, I gave careful thought as to what descriptive designation is most suitable for the person whom this publication will assist and I came to the conclusion that the most appropriate word is *athlete*. The definition in the Oxford Dictionary of this word is 'competitor or skilled performer in physical exercises; robust or vigorous person'. This seems to be a very apt interpretation; therefore the word has been used throughout this book in the generic sense.

Rex Hazeldine

CHAPTER 1
An Understanding of Fitness

PHYSICAL FITNESS

Terms such as 'physical fitness', 'physical training' and 'conditioning' are used in various ways by educationists, sports scientists, coaches and athletes, yet the way in which these terms are related is often unclear. In order to clarify the definitions of these terms and to help with understanding the total concept of physical fitness, a model is presented in Fig. 1. By working from a model of this kind, you are encouraged to take a more balanced approach to increasing levels of fitness through being made aware of the contribution of the various components to the total state of physical fitness.

Physical fitness as a term refers to the total dynamic physiological state of the individual, ranging on a continuum from optimal human performance to severe debilitation and death. Athletes would be found towards the upper end of the continuum, fluctuating up or down depending on their state of training, whilst at the other end conditions of illness could exist.

While the term 'fitness' may be satisfactory in a descriptive sense, problems arise when attempts are made to define the concept in an operational way, that is when we try to measure or develop it. The complexity arises because fitness is made up of a series of components such as strength, endurance,

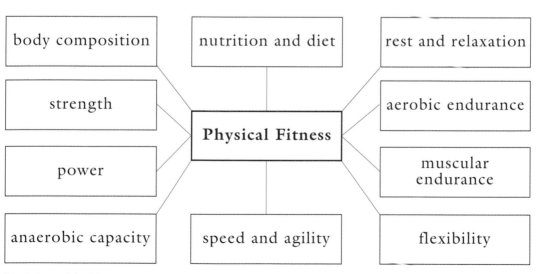

Fig 1 A model of fitness.

flexibility and so on, each of which makes some independent contribution to the whole state *(Fig 1)*. While some of the components are related, it is possible for an athlete to have a great deal of one component and very little of another. Also, when considering the wide range of sports, certain components assume a considerable importance; the necessity for flexibility in gymnastics, the importance of strength and power in weight-lifting and the quality of endurance in marathon running. Most sports, of course, require a contribution from several of the components of fitness, in varying degrees.

Physical Training or Conditioning

Physical training or conditioning refers to the processes used in order to develop the components of physical fitness such as how to improve aerobic endurance, to stretch and relax muscles, to increase arm and shoulder strength, and to relate exercises and programmes to the specific requirements of individual sports.

Body Composition

Body composition refers to the proportions of lean body mass and body fat. It is more important than total weight as a component of physical fitness, since it is possible for a very muscular person to be overweight according to popular height-weight tables, and still have a relatively small percentage of weight deposited as fat.

Aerobic Endurance

Aerobic endurance refers to prolonged activity of low intensity indicating the capacity to continue physical work and withstand the onset of fatigue.

Muscular Endurance

Muscular endurance is the capacity of a muscle or group of muscles to do work continuously.

Anaerobic Capacity

Anaerobic capacity is the total amount of energy which can be supplied by anaerobic metabolism.

Flexibility

Flexibility is the range of movement at a joint or at joint complexes.

Speed

Speed refers to the time taken to co-ordinate joint actions or to transport the whole body through space.

Agility

Agility is the ability to stop, start and change direction of body movements in short periods of time.

Strength

Strength is the force that a muscle or group of muscles can generate against a resistance.

Power

Power is the combination of speed (velocity) and strength to produce explosive movements.

WARM-UP AND COOL-DOWN

In addition to understanding the concept of physical fitness, and adopting a balanced approach to improving your state of fitness, it is important to develop and adopt sensible *training habits* towards fitness training.

The first habit is the desirability of adequately warming-up and cooling-down. During physical training or competition, the physiological systems of the body are working to adapt to exercise-induced stress. Therefore, it is advisable to warm up in preparation for the increased energy demands which muscles and related systems have to cope with during exercise or performance. Essentially, warm-up decreases the chances of injury by raising the muscle temperature, increasing blood flow and by stretching muscles, ligaments and connective tissue; improves physical efficiency and prepares the body for work by raising the heart, metabolic and respiratory rates. Demands are made gradually and progressively on the circulatory and respiratory systems, so that little or no discomfort may be felt. In many situations, warm-up contains careful rehearsal of skill patterns involved in the actual performance.

Guidelines for Warm-Up

1. Adopt a whole-body warm-up which raises muscle and blood temperature, and which gradually increases heart-rate – light running is an example of this kind of activity.
2. Carefully stretch muscles and connective tissue. All the main joints should be worked by concentrating on any muscle groups to be used in the 'performance.

3. Use related warm-up, so that any practice effect may be achieved simultaneously.
4. Warm-up should be suited to both the athlete and activity.
5. Your warm-up should be a combination of intensity and duration without undue fatigue.
6. Avoid time-lag between warm-up and competition/training.

Cool-Down

Most athletes appreciate the need to warm-up, but often seem unaware of the values of a cool-down. When the period of exertion is over, many adaptations have to be made during the process of recovery before the body returns to normal. The recovery process will take some time, but the body can be helped in the very earliest stage to clear waste products and the general aftermath of exertion. The muscles which have been helping to pump the blood back to the heart are no longer active, and there is a build-up of pressure in the muscle which results in the accumulation of excess body tissue fluid. This condition, with inadequate muscle forces to move the blood out of the muscle, may result in subsequent stiffness or soreness. Generally, the adaptations which the body has to bring about in the recovery phase can be helped by mild rhythmic-type muscular activity, gradually decreasing in intensity, and some stretching until a near resting state is reached. Hot showers, baths or massage will generally help the recovery process.

CHAPTER 2
Introduction to Training

ENERGY SYSTEMS *(Fig 2)*

For muscular work of any type to take place, energy is required. The immediate source of energy in the muscle is an energy rich compound called *adenosine triphosphate* (ATP). There are three energy systems in the human body which produce ATP for muscular contraction.

1. The stored, starting up energy system, uses another energy rich compound *phosphocreatine* (PC), which combines with ADP to produce energy. No oxygen is required for this system, so it can be called anaerobic.
2. The breakdown of stored carbohydrates in the absence of oxygen supplies the energy for muscular contraction (the re-synthesis of ATP). The carbohydrate which is used is either stored glycogen (a storage form of glucose), circulating blood glucose, or glycogen stored in the liver, which is converted to glucose and then enters the bloodstream to be carried to the muscles. This again is an anaerobic system, and in this case lactic acid is produced.
3. The breakdown of stored carbohydrates and fats in the presence of oxygen (an aerobic system) supplies the energy for muscular contraction. The carbohydrate comes from the same sources previously described, glycogen in the muscle, circulating blood glucose and liver glycogen, and the fats come from the adipose sites, and to a lesser extent from fat globules found in the muscle cell.

The muscles are made up of a mixture of fibres, of two distinct types:

1. The fast twitch, quick-sprint type which contract rapidly but fatigue easily.
2. The slow twitch, longer running type which contract slowly but keep going longer.

The fast twitch muscle fibres are responsible for the high speed movements, but for short periods of time. They use carbohydrate for 'fuel' and produce lactic acid which, as it builds up gradually, inhibits the muscle contracting.

The slow-twitch muscle fibres produce less power, but can continue for longer periods of time. They work at a lower level of effort, use a combination of carbohydrate and fat burned in the presence of oxygen, and the main waste product in this case is carbon dioxide, which can be easily removed from the body.

The athlete's body is capable of using just one, or any combination of the three energy systems. Different sports demand different types and amounts of muscular activity. Consequently, different energy systems are brought into play, and the type of muscle fibres used will determine which energy system will be used. If we take the simple example of any athlete starting to run, in the first few seconds, the ATP-PC system will make the main contribution to producing the energy required, as the creatine phosphate is there ready in the muscle. The second system, using

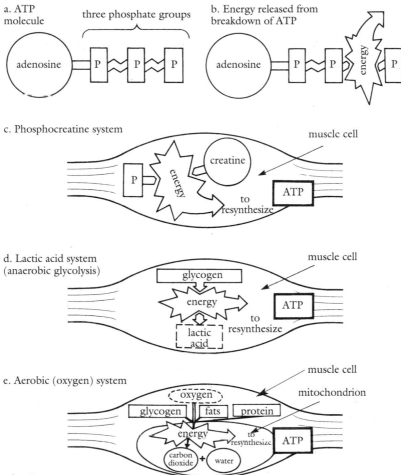

Fig 2 Energy systems.

glycogen and converting it to ATP, called *gly-colysis*, will also contribute from the start, but it will take time going 'through the gears', with the chemical reactions taking place to break down the glycogen. The third system, the aerobic system, will also contribute with the small amount of oxygen stored in the muscle, but there will be a little delay in the cardio-vascular system supplying the oxygen at the required rate in the very early stages. As the running becomes more prolonged, the aerobic system will make the main contribution as it is the most efficient system, able to use the full range of stored energy and without the inhibiting effects of lactic acid.

The degree of involvement of the energy systems will further depend on the nature and intensity of the activity. Consider two contrasting activities; the sprinter will depend mainly on anaerobic energy using fast twitch fibres. The ATP-PC will be used because it is there, immediate and ready; the second system, using glycolysis, will be used predominantly because it can supply energy at a very high rate. The marathon runner will produce most of the energy using the aerobic system and the slow twitch fibres. The marathon runner, though, will have to run at a pace that will allow the cardio-vascular system to supply oxygen at a rate which will match the demand.

The games player will use a combination of different energy systems and, as the activity in games is usually intermittent, with intervals of work and intervals of rest, the games player will have to recover from hard bouts of work, and is given the chance to replenish some of the energy stores and remove the inhibitory waste products.

FATIGUE

What causes fatigue? What prevents an athlete from working at his or her maximal capacity for unlimited periods of time? The answer to these questions can be simplified by identifying two causes, firstly running out of 'fuel', and secondly inhibitory effects.

Running out of fuel refers to:

1. Size of the stores:
    (a) the phosphagens; the total muscular stores of ATP and PC.
    (b) glycogen; the form in which carbohydrate is stored in the body.
Some oxygen is bound to the myoglobin in the muscle.
2. Rate of utilization; the rate at which ATP is required and used.
3. Rate of repletion; the rate at which the refuelling takes place.

Inhibitory effects refer to the accumulation of products which have an inhibitory effect on muscle function, causing it to slow down and not work as efficiently. Mainly this relates to the end products of glycolysis, particularly lactic acid.

If the body could build up a store of ATP in the muscle this could be used as the available fuel, but this is not the case. Only trace amounts of ATP are stored in the muscle cells and the body has to produce ATP at the rate at which it is required. The previous section on energy systems described how the body regenerates ATP from the stores of phosphocreatine, glycogen and fat. At the onset and during any activity all systems will make a contribution to energy provision but at a different rate dependent on time and the intensity of the activity. Short bouts of very intensive effort will predominantly use phosphocreatine, because of its availability, and glycogen which is converted to lactic acid producing ATP at a fast rate without requiring oxygen. During the rest intervals in intermittent activity, characteristic of games like hockey, the body is given some opportunity to refuel, i.e. to replenish to a certain extent the phosphocreatine stores to be used again in the subsequent intervals of work.

With high level bursts of work like sprinting, fatigue is detectable after 20 seconds. Muscle glycogen stores could provide ATP for at least 70 to 80 seconds of all-out sprinting. Measurements on the muscles of athletes exhausted by a bout of sprinting show that some glycogen is still present in the muscles, so in this kind of activity one can look for the main cause of fatigue from the inhibitory effects of the accumulation of the end products of glycolysis.

Lactic Acid

The build up of lactic acid in the muscle will tend to have two basic effects – *enzyme inhibition* which slows down the whole process of glycolysis and thus the production of ATP from this source, and *mechanical impairment* where the actual process of muscular contraction is eventually interfered with, reducing the power output of the muscle.

As the intensity of effort, or speed of the runner, increases towards maximum aerobic capacity, the body becomes more dependent on anaerobic glycolysis with an increase in the production of lactic acid. Training should enable an athlete to run closer to his or her maximal aerobic capacity, in some cases at 80 to 90 per cent, without producing lactic acid; this means that the ATP requirement is being met by the aerobic system. The trained athlete also appears to have an increased capacity to tolerate, and an increased ability to remove, lactic acid.

PRINCIPLES OF TRAINING

There are some basic guidelines which need to be considered when designing effective fitness programmes.

Intensity

For any of the body systems to improve, it must be stressed or made to work harder than it does normally – the principle is called *overload*. By intensity is meant the level at which the system is overloaded. The amount of overload influences the rate at which the physiological adaptations take place. As a general rule, the greater the intensity, the greater the physiological improvement in the particular system being worked. Below a certain stress level, the athlete will at best merely maintain a current level of fitness. The intensity which produces optimal physiological adaptation will vary according to the system being exercised and the fitness level of the athlete.

Duration

This refers to the amount of time necessary within a single bout of training, to provide sufficient overload to a particular system to encourage the optimal physiological adaptations. It will again vary with the fitness level of the athlete and the system being stressed.

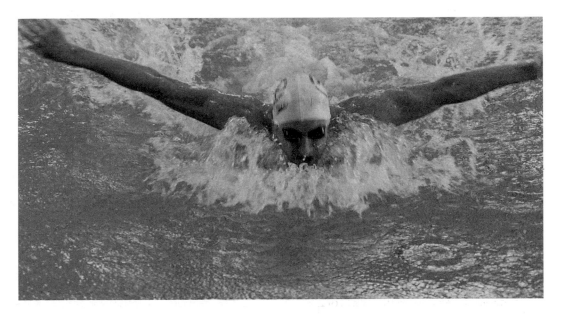

Fig 3 International swimmer in training.

Frequency

This denotes the number of sessions per week, per month, per year. After a particular system has been overloaded, it needs rest to allow the body to adapt and rebuild the system to a higher physiological level than before. Again, this varies between individuals and according to the nature of the training programme.

Progression

Training programmes should be planned so that the loads are increased to provide slow steady progress, which will enable the desired adaptations to take place in the right way. This is helped by keeping a record of training, so that sensible progression can be built into the system.

Specificity

Training programmes should be devised and geared to the specific demands of the sport or activity. The starting point is an evaluation of the sport in order to establish the particular systems concerned, and the way in which these systems are required to operate. For instance, one sport may require steady, prolonged effort, whilst another sport may demand numerous short bursts of intensive activity, interspersed with frequent periods of rest. *Preparation must be tailored to suit these particular demands.* In order to do this the concept of physiological specificity needs to be understood. If the training involves steady-state, low-intensity effort the result will be an increase in endurance with little or no effect on speed and strength.

Conversely, sprint training should increase running speed, but will have little effect on endurance.

Training is essentially about adaptation *(Fig 4)*. The actual training session provides a challenge to the body, a stress which causes the body to make adaptations in the period following the training in order to cope with another challenge. The adaptations which take place depend on the nature of the stress. If it is endurance training the body becomes more efficient at providing energy aerobically; if weight training, there is an increase in the size and strength of muscle fibres and connective tissue.

Variation

Training needs to be long term to achieve any worthwhile physiological adaptations, so there is a real danger of boredom and monotony. Athletes have to accept the discipline of training, but where possible it is important to vary the exercises and training routines in order to maintain motivation and to stimulate interest.

Reversibility

Most of the physiological adaptations which result from hard training are reversible; fitness is hard to gain but easy to lose. Long term planning of training programmes, although there may be different phases in intensity, should ensure that long periods of inactivity are provided. If illness, or injury, forces inactivity on the athlete, it must be accepted that resumption of training will begin at a lower level.

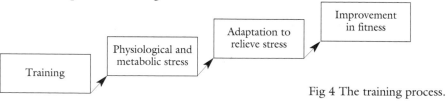

Fig 4 The training process.

STRUCTURING THE TRAINING

This section outlines the principles and methods for structuring a programme of training. Each programme will be different in terms of age and sex of athlete, availability of time and facilities, and level of performance, so it is not possible to be too specific. But, based on a knowledge of the components of physical fitness, previously outlined in the text, an understanding of the relevance and contribution of the various areas in the extensive range of physical performance, a knowledge of basic principles and planning should provide the means to design a training programme adapted to the needs of an athlete or a team of athletes. This kind of approach, rather than accepting and following slavishly the prescriptions of others, can promote more meaningful development in fitness training for sport.

Analysis

Firstly, it is necessary to analyse the relevance of the contribution of fitness and training theory to the extensive range of sports performance and to appreciate that fitness for sport is fundamentally the capacity to delay the onset of fatigue since this will adversely affect performance in a number of possible ways, such as low work rate, deterioration in technique, and poor judgement. Fitness training for sport needs to be a constant search for the link between training and performance. The starting point is an *evaluation* of the requirements of the sport, and in the context of games, the particular positional needs of the player which should provide the necessary information for selecting *relevant* training methods and types of exercises. These elements are then organized into a programme and the overall process is one of progressive adaptation.

Structure

The training programme is structured to provide divisions in the total training which vary in duration and the nature and intensity of the training prescription practised in each phase. To be on a sound physiological basis, training should be planned on a cyclical year-long process *(Fig 5)* which is part of a long-term progression of training. In putting the programme together, the divisions which can be used are:

1. Preparation; two phases.
   (a) Out-of-season – emphasis on general training as a basis for specialized and competition-based training.
   (b) Pre-season – training specifically related to the demands of the sport and the athlete's level of development.
2. Competition; the retention of levels of fitness, preparation for vital performances and coping with injury, illness and the stresses of competition.
3. Recuperation; transition from competition to the start of the out-of-season phase of preparation.

Preparation: Out-of-Season Phase

Most athletes of good standard recognize the value of maintaining physical fitness during the

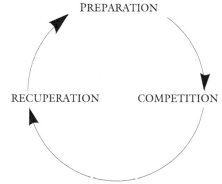

Fig 5 The cycle of training.

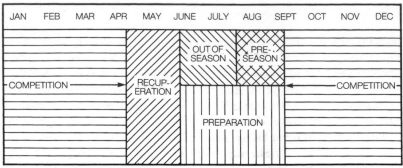

Fig 6 An example of a year-round training programme – rugby football.

out-of-season phase. Maintenance and development of certain levels and qualities of fitness provide a logical preparation for the more intensive pre-season training. The out-of-season stage is also an ideal time for overcoming previously exposed limitations and weaknesses.

This phase is an ideal time to concentrate on aerobic training. Time is available for the continuous type of training which is an effective means of developing a sound 'aerobic base', the foundation required for other forms of training to follow. There will be concentration on continuous submaxial exercise, such as long continuous running, and training will be high in extent and low in intensity. Methods of training such as fartlek (*see* page 23) can be used for variety. Since the athlete is not engaged in regular competition, this is a suitable time for strength training. Emphasis should be on using exercises which employ all the major muscle groups; squats, cleans and bench press are applicable illustrations for this type of work, to serve as a base in a similar way to aerobic training for the more specific strength work later. Flexibility work can usefully be included throughout all phases of the training programme, progressively moving from the general to the specific.

Preparation: Pre-Season Phase

If the out-of-season programmes are conducted properly, pre-season training can be designed to bring the athlete to a high level of fitness in the shortest possible time. The intensity of the aerobic training can be increased by progressively introducing interval training. The programme at this stage will include exercises to improve muscular endurance, anaerobic capacity and develop speed. The main gain of the pre-season strength is preparation to meet the demands of the sport, so strength training will change emphasis from general strength work to more specialized strength exercises. Strength must be usable at the speed of the sport. Strength training sessions should be designed to develop forces under optimal speeds and repetitions to facilitate increases in speed and endurance while maintaining basic strength. If applicable, plyometrics (*see* page 102) can be used effectively at this stage. Often less time is available for strength training for many sports during the pre-season phase because of the need to concentrate on skills and strategy.

Competition

Physical fitness levels are reversible, although it is true that it takes less time to maintain an improved fitness level than it does to attain it. Too many athletes abandon serious physical training once the competition phase is underway for reasons of lack of time, other priorities or an attitude that training is now unnecessary. The athlete who has trained seriously and progressively through the preparation phase does face the prospect of some regression during the competition phase. This will vary with the

18

nature of the sport, but it will be more marked in the less demanding activities.

Aerobic training can be maintained for most sports on one or two sessions per week. This refers to maintaining a level of aerobic fitness generally, not to the particular demands of sports with a significant endurance factor. Long, easy-paced runs may be used as light but active recovery from the heavy demands of matches and more strenuous training, or they could form the basis of a long warm-up prior to practice or fitness sessions. Anaerobic training should be maintained at levels achieved in the pre-season and even increased in those sports which require a high anaerobic capacity. The main objectives of the competition phase strength training are to maintain levels of specialized strength, develop new levels of competition based strength, and help prevention of injury. Athletes who are capable of increasing resistance during this phase should do so gradually, ensuring that speed or endurance, if required, are not sacrificed. If the areas of the body most subject to injury are given some attention, and strength is maintained in the related muscle groups, this can help to reduce the risk of injury. As with aerobic training, strength levels can be maintained by far less work than is required to obtain peak levels. For most sports, other than those demanding significant strength qualities, one or two training sessions per week should be sufficient.

During this phase any particular main competition, climax or a number of associated main competitions bring their own special demands. A particular phase of application has to be designed which will require a planned 'blending' of training methods and intensities prior to building for the peak level desired for which the timing of the assault will be a vital factor.

Recuperation

Most athletes regard the end of a long competitive season as the start of a lengthy period of rest and relaxation. A full recovery from the rigours of the competition phase is necessary in order to provide maximum potential for the next cycle of training. The recuperation phase should involve a *gradual* reduction in all forms of training rather than a sudden withdrawal, and a transition to lighter more relaxing activities which also have the desired psychological effects and, importantly, avoid total abstinence from physical activity.

Contra-Indicated Exercises

In planning a training programme, you should give attention to the possible dangers of certain exercises. Some exercises used routinely in training could be harmful to the participants, for example, for years straight leg 'trunk curls' and 'leg raises' have been used to strengthen the abdomen muscles. Unfortunately, these exercises make particular use of the psoas and iliacus muscles (two of the hip flexors) rather than the abdominal muscles. The psoas muscle attaches directly to the interior portions of the lumbar spine, so that the forceful contraction may result in hyperextension of the lower back, particularly if the abdominal muscles are relatively weak which is often the case. When the body is in the supine position, as for trunk curls, the psoas muscle tends to hyperextend the lower back and iliacus causes the pelvis to tilt forward. If the abdominals contract simultaneously, the forward tilt of the pelvis may be prevented and hip flexion occurs. But, if the abdominal muscles are weak, the lumbar vertebrae are raised off the floor and iliopsoas muscles perform the major part of the movement with the abdominal muscles merely assisting isometrically to stabilize the pelvis. Lower back problems could result from this kind of exercise. A recommended substitute for 'trunk curls' is the 'abdominal curl' with the knees *bent*.

Another danger area is the stress which deep knee squats and 'bounces' in this position exert on the knee joint. The knee is a weight-bearing joint and is considerably stressed in a number of sports, which is demonstrated by the high incidence of injury. The stability of the joint and ligaments are put under considerable strain in the deep squat position, and it is recommended in most cases to avoid lowering the body past an angle of 90 degrees at the joint. This is particularly important in weight training where heavy loads may be used. In this context, the spine is also vulnerable, so the emphasis is always on a sound and safe technique. There are other examples of questionable exercises which indicate that athletes should give careful consideration to the analysis of anatomical and mechanical principles associated with selected exercises.

Careful evaluation, selection of exercises and methods of training, planning and structuring of loadings, awareness of potential injury, use of a comprehensive and balanced fitness programme are essential for the development and realization of potential in any sport.

THE YOUNGER ATHLETE

Training prescriptions for young athletes should give consideration to the fact that, although children between nine and sixteen years of age are at their most adaptable physiologically, they need to expend considerable energy in growing and maturing. In addition, there is a certain amount of fragility in the structural and functional changes which are part of the growth process. Although carefully selected and monitored strength training, using body resistance exercises, can be used, any heavy weight training certainly should not until near the completion of growth, in most cases after sixteen or seventeen years of age. Similarly, anaerobic type work should not be emphasized in the early years, but flexibility, which

will begin to decline after nine or ten years of age, can be usefully employed to maintain the peak levels evident in that age group.

Endurance can best be developed through simple running sports, orienteering and attractive forms of cross-country running, together with various field games.

In all forms of training with young children, strict consideration should be given to the balance between carefully evaluated intervals of work and adequate rest periods.

THE OLDER ATHLETE

With older athletes, it should be borne in mind that the physiological effects of regular exercise and training are not appreciably different with age. The same benefits can be experienced by individuals of any age. In fact, with the older athlete who may have suffered physical deterioration due to years of inactivity, exercise can be positively beneficial in, for example, weight control and to combat obesity, possibly keeping arthritic joints lubricated and improving the efficiency of the heart.

But, with regard to the planning of training with the older athlete who may have suffered physical deterioration due to years of inactivity, exercise can be positively beneficial in, for example, weight control and to combat obesity, possibly keeping arthritic joints lubricated and improving the efficiency of the heart.

But, with regard to the planning of training programmes, it must be accepted that the older athlete is likely to be more unfit than the younger counterpart, that the physiological adaptations to training take place more slowly, that his/her maximum capacities (aerobic capacity and heart rate, for example) will be lower, that the likelihood of some cardiac problem is increased, that there will be a greater susceptibility to injury and normally a longer time needed for recovery.

CHAPTER 3
Endurance

There are two kinds of endurance: *aerobic endurance* refers to the process of taking in, transporting and using oxygen, whilst *muscular endurance* represents the capacity of the muscle for continuous performance of localized activity. They are, of course, inter-related.

AEROBIC ENDURANCE

The lungs, heart and blood vessels perform a vital function as the body's supply system. They supply the muscles with the necessary fuels and oxygen, and carry away waste products such as carbon dioxide and lactic acid. Consequently, the cardio-respiratory system in the athlete needs to be developed to match the muscles which it supplies and cleanses. Aerobic capacity, known by the abbreviation VO_2max, is a physiological parameter much measured by sports scientists, and is the maximum volume of oxygen which can be used per minute by an individual. It is measured in litres per minute, but as there is variation in body size between individuals it is usually reported per kilogram of body weight. Endurance training should increase an athlete's aerobic capacity ($\dot{V}O_2$max), and it is known that trained

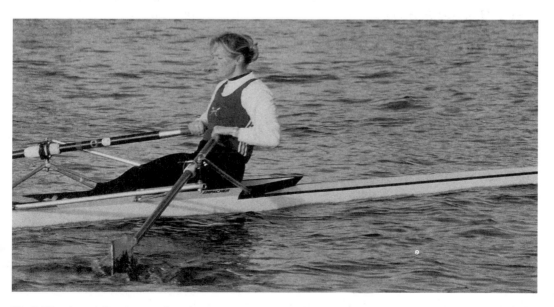

Fig 7 The demanding sport of rowing.

endurance male athletes can have high aerobic capacities of 60/70ml per kg compared to an average figure for a twenty-year-old male of 45ml per kg.

Certain sports (marathon running is a good illustration) will require high levels of aerobic endurance, but it can be recommended as a desirable quality for almost all athletes to have a good aerobic base. Many sports, such as games, require prolonged effort and a considerable amount of running, although these may be intermittent, and on a sound foundation of aerobic endurance other fitness qualities can be more effectively developed.

Aerobic Training

Three types of aerobic training, using the activity of running, can be employed to develop aerobic capacity. Where suitable and applicable, similar training systems can be used with other activities, i.e. the use of interval training by swimmers.

Long Continuous Running

This is fundamental to so many sports, and can be referred to as the base of a pyramid; the larger the base (the greater the duration and number of runs), the greater is the potential for improvement of the other body systems. Jogging, as it is called in some situations, is a suitable beginning for most people. Regular training of this kind makes the lungs work more effectively, allowing more air to reach the blood as it is pumped through the lungs. It also increases the capacity of the blood to carry the oxygen and deliver it to the muscles. This form of steady exercise produces a gradual increase in the working capacity of the heart, which is reflected in a drop in the pulse rate. As training progresses it can be noted that pulse rate, providing a simple indication

of the heart rate, will be lower at the same work load during exercise, indicating a more efficient cardio-vascular response, and pulse rate at rest could be lower. The increased pressure on the circulatory system can also open up under-developed blood vessels and develop new capillaries (very small blood vessels) in the muscles, which will provide a more efficient blood circulation to and from the muscles.

Someone beginning training who has not been a regular exerciser could have a low oxygen uptake, so in the early stages this should be improved by means of gentle exercise at the aerobic level. Increased effort too rapidly changes the aerobic state into an anaerobic state; lactic acid builds up in the muscles leading rapidly to muscular fatigue. Progression is the key, beginning with small distances and low intensities of effort. Eventually, a standard training run could be two to five miles, but naturally it must vary with the state of fitness by the athlete. Endurance athletes will use large amounts of long continuous running.

One way to approach long continuous running is to do a series of runs over a measured distance and time each run, gradually attempting to reduce the time. It could be carried out in the form of a circuit equivalent to about one mile. As the running becomes easier, the distance should be increased, while simultaneously trying to reduce the time. You might start with an average of an eight minute/mile pace over two miles. Six weeks later you might be running five miles at an average seven minute/mile pace. Another method is to commence at a steady pace, and run from a particular point for a specified length of time, possibly fifteen minutes. The distance run should then be increased, while the time remains the same.

The heart rate is a good indicator for controlling the intensity of exercise. A suggested level is between 130 and 160 beats per minute for at least thirty minutes.

It is useful during many forms of exercise to measure heart rate to give an indication of intensity of effort. This can be done simply by taking the pulse (radial pulse). To do this, place fingers on the underside of the wrist in line with the base of the thumb. Count the number of beats for fifteen seconds and then multiply by four to give an estimate of heart rate per minute.

Varied Pace Running

A combination of aerobic and anaerobic endurance is accomplished in a varied pace run by interrupting steady, continuous running with occasional faster running or short sprints. The forced entry into periods of anaerobic work, and consequent oxygen debt during the fast pace, demands repayment during the following phase of easy running. This situation acts as a stimulus for the improvement of maximum oxygen uptake and speed recovery. It is designed to improve endurance qualities, and the ability of the athlete to tolerate and recover from the effects of running at faster speeds. The method is most applicable to the running demands of field games.

One established form of varied pace running is known as *fartlek*. It is a Swedish word meaning 'speed play', and was originally intended as a refresher amid repetitive, tightly controlled work on the athletics track. Although it is not vital to run in the natural surroundings of hills, forests, fields or sands, a varied terrain with inclines and soft surfaces provides a most suitable environment for this form of training. Notwithstanding the fact that the athlete usually determines the length and timing of intermittent changes in pace, fartlek running should not be treated as a carefree method of training. It should be planned precisely to create overload situations with appropriate recovery phases.

A typical fartlek session (30 minutes) could be:

1. Jogging (5 minutes).
2. A fast evenly paced run (3 minutes).
3. Brisk walk (2 minutes).
4. Evenly paced running with 50–60 metre sprints every 200 metres (5 minutes).
5. Jogging (2 minutes).
6. Evenly paced running with occasional inclusion of four/five fast strides, small acceleration sprints (3 minutes).
7. Jogging with one fast uphill run (20–30 metres) in every minute (5 minutes).
8. Jogging and rhythmical exercises, skipping and gentle knee raises (5 minutes).

Interval Running

Interval running consists of running a specified number of distances (from 100 to 1,000 metres) in a given time, with short recoveries or rest periods. The basis for interval running programmes is that when bouts of heavy work are interspersed with short rest periods, the total work load can be greatly increased beyond that which might be achieved during a single continuous bout at the same intensity of work. Interval running is more effectively introduced after general cardio-respiratory fitness has been developed by long continuous and varied paced running. Depending on the nature of the programme, interval running has the potential of improving both aerobic and anaerobic capacity. The latter quality can be developed by increasing the intensity of the work, in order to place greater demands on the oxidative capacity of the muscles. This requires fast running for distances long enough to ensure that the athlete is thoroughly fatigued near the completion of the run. This will cause an oxygen debt, accompanied by a build-up of lactic acid in the muscle, and then in the blood, which will stimulate oxidative adaptations. This form of training will have an effect on lung and heart function, and on the athlete's aerobic capacity. As with all forms of training, the physiological adaptations will relate to the nature and intensity of the programme. Effective use of the interval running method involves the manipulation of certain factors:

1. Length of the work interval – the longer the work interval, the more endurance factors are involved. Distances will be selected which are appropriate to the requirements of the particular sport. Completion of intervals longer than competitive distances is especially useful in the out of season, preparatory phase to help develop an aerobic base.

2. Pace of the runs – this can be measured in two ways, either by running at a certain level of effort, or by running at a certain pace. The two methods are obviously related, but in the first the approach is to establish a level of effort by obtaining a maximum for the distance, say 50 seconds for 300 metres; and then the athlete runs the 300 metres at 90 per cent effort in 55 seconds: or 80 per cent effort in 60 seconds. In this way, the intensity of the effort can be controlled for each run for the individual athlete. The second method simply requires the athlete to repeat intervals at the same speed, say 600 metres in 1 minute 30 seconds, or at varying pace by progressively increasing or decreasing the pace, or by alternating fast and slow intervals.

3. Number of repetitions – the number of work intervals will depend on many factors; the condition of the athlete, the training period, the particular sport and the physiological adaptations sought, but the number will be related to intensity, and the nearer an athlete is to maximum effort, then the fewer there need be.

4. Length of rest intervals – again, the length of the rest intervals between repetitions depends on the system the athlete is trying to develop. To start with, the recovery period should be of sufficient length for an athlete to feel that he can run the next work interval as fast as the previous one. A heart-rate value (using pulse counts as described) of 100 to 120 beats per minute is usual before continuing. Shortening the rest interval and making the work interval less intense, will make the training more effective in terms of endurance. Increasing the rest interval (within certain limits) and intensifying the work interval, will develop speed qualities more effectively.

5. Form of rest – athletes should be encouraged to jog or walk briskly during the rest interval, as some form of light exercise will help the clearance of lactic acid and other waste products, thus producing a better recovery.

ANAEROBIC CAPACITY

Many sports involve bursts of high-intensity effort when a large amount of energy is required very rapidly. The aerobic system cannot supply sufficient energy during these phases so a significant amount of energy is supplied from anaerobic systems. One of these energy systems breaks down stored carbohydrates (glycogen) to produce energy quickly, but one of the end-products is lactic acid which, as it builds up in the muscle, is a major cause of fatigue. As previously explained, this build-up of lactate has two main effects: 'enzyme inhibition' which slows down the process of glycolysis and thus the provision of energy from this source; and 'mechanical impairment' which interferes with contraction of the muscles, thus reducing the power output of the muscle. Training is required which helps the athlete cope with this build-up of lactic acid in the muscles and also helps to disperse the lactate more quickly and efficiently.

The type of training needed is 'short interval work' or shuttle running, which helps the athlete tolerate the effects of bouts of high intensity work and recover more rapidly.

1. Athletes can 'work' for a set time interval of 30 seconds interspersed with 30 seconds' rest. This can be sprinting or some sport-specific activity.
2. Similarly, athletes can work for a set time interval of 40 seconds with a 20 seconds' interval.

Shuttle Running

Shuttle running is a widely used training method to improve sprint explosiveness and the ability to recover from maximal or near maximal bouts of work. The system imitates a situation found especially in the games area where series of intensive effort are interspersed with intervals of rest.

Possible Schedules

1. Work in pairs for set time intervals of 60 to 100 seconds with intervals of rest of 20 seconds. Partners *alternate* sprinting to a line ten or fifteen or twenty metres away and sprinting back.
2. Work in pairs for set time intervals of 30 to 60 seconds. One partner shuttle runs a set distance (ten to twenty metres) for 30 seconds, then rests for the same time interval, whilst the other partner runs.
3. Work in pairs for set time interval of 30 to 60 seconds. One partner shuttle runs to a distance of ten metres, then fifteen metres, then twenty metres and repeats the sequence for the interval of work, then rests for the same time interval whilst the other partner shuttle runs.

MUSCULAR ENDURANCE

Muscular endurance represents the capacity of the athlete for continuous performance of relatively heavy localized activity which may make only small demands on the functions of respiration and circulation before exhaustion sets in. The more often a muscle performs a movement in training, over the same range, against the same resistance, and at the same frequency and speed as required in competition, then the less likely it is to become locally fatigued by that movement during competition. The improvement is primarily due to the functional involvement of more muscle fibres (motor units) as a result of overload. Overload also improves the utilization of oxygen by involving more capillaries, thus providing the working muscles with more oxygen and fuel, as well as facilitating the removal of the metabolic waste products of strenuous exercise.

CIRCUIT TRAINING

Circuit training is a widely used and proven method of improving muscular endurance and, dependent on the type of circuit used, it has been shown to produce positive changes in general fitness, muscular strength and speed.

There are many variations of circuit training, but most methods employ the following factors: the progressive resistance exercises; the use of body resistance and/or apparatus exercises; a circular arrangement of the exercises which permits progression from one station to another until all stations have been visited, the total comprising a circuit; a limiting time factor within which the circuit must be concluded, or a certain prescription of exercises. From these factors the following should be considered:

1. Between eight and fifteen different exercise stations is most usual, and innumerable exercises and exercise variations can be included in the circuit. Each exercise should be selected for its potential in developing certain qualities, be it a component of general fitness or a specific requirement associated with a sport. In addition, the variety of exercises should provide a balanced loading on different body parts.

2. The sequence of exercises should be organized to avoid, as far as possible, two consecutive stations stressing the same muscle groups. This should encourage active local recovery of the worked muscles, whilst an accumulative load is maintained on the heart, lungs and circulatory system.

3. Many of the exercises will employ body weight as resistance, which can be varied as described in the chapter on strength. But weights, ropes, medicine balls and other equipment are used as further types of resistance. The level of resistance used will be dependent on the kind of adaptation required.

4. The resistance and type of exercise used should be adjusted so that the working muscles are capable of performing as many repetitions as possible within the specified work interval (e.g. 60 seconds) with noticeable fatigue on completion. Once one circuit (a set of exercises) has been completed, it is possible to add further sets to provide a more demanding schedule.

5. The physiological processes involved during the recovery period are as important as the energy processes involved during the work itself, consequently, the selection of an appropriate rest or recovery interval is essential in the organization of an effective circuit. Variations in the length of the rest interval related to the length of the work interval will change the emphasis on the energy systems being used, and thus the type of fitness being developed.

6. It is possible to record the number of repetitions achieved in a certain time, or the time taken to achieve a set number of repetitions. Target time limits can be designated for the completion of a circuit. This recording of information can help to monitor progress, and provide a degree of motivation. Progression can be implemented through increase in work interval, reduction of recovery interval – and introduction of second and third circuits.

Circuit training can have wide-ranging influences including the needs of the beginner, the improvement of general fitness and the specific needs of the different sports. A gymnasium with its equipment is a very suitable environment, but a circuit can be adopted for most outdoor and indoor spaces. Moreover, it is a form of training which is economical on time.

A basic knowledge of the factors which govern the organization of circuit training should enable the design of a routine of exercises suited to any training purpose. To provide some familiarization with the application of this knowledge, a number of circuits are outlined in the following section.

FITNESS CIRCUITS

Circuit A – General Fitness Circuit

Circuit A is an example of a general fitness circuit, with a minimum of equipment, which could be used as an introduction to this form of training or developed for improvement of general fitness.

1. *Push-up (Fig 8)* Front support position with arms shoulder width apart: arms bend to lower the chest to the floor and return to front support position; keep a rigid body throughout (this can be made easier by adopting the kneeling position).

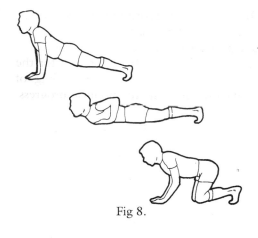

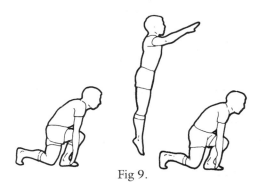

Fig 8.

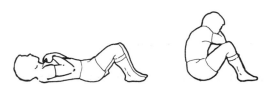

Fig 9.

2. *Vertical jump (Fig 9)* From position of kneeling on one leg with fingers touching floor, jump up and change legs to land in opposite kneeling position.

3. *Abdominal curl (Fig 10)* Lie on back with knees bent and hands across the chest: raise trunk and touch both knees with both elbows: for the next repetition, touch left knee with right elbow, next the right knee with left elbow: then back to straight abdominal curl: keep up this rotation exercising in three directions.

4. *Back extension (Fig 11)* Lie on front with feet fixed (under bench or wall-bars): slowly raise trunk off the floor and gently lower.

5. *Astride jumping over bench (Fig 12)* Stand astride a bench or other suitable platform: jump with both feet to stand on bench and then jump back to stand astride in original starting position. Repeat rhythmically and continuously.

6. *Pull-up (Fig 13)* Overgrasp or undergrasp on a beam or bar: pull up to touch beam/bar with chin, then lower to full elbow extension (this can be made easier by having feet on floor and adopting an angled position).

7. *Bench stepping (Fig 14)* Step on and off a chair or bench: ensure that legs and back are perfectly straight when both feet are on chair/bench.

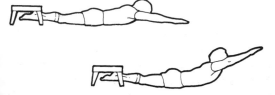

Fig 10.

Fig 11.

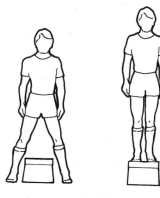

Fig 12.

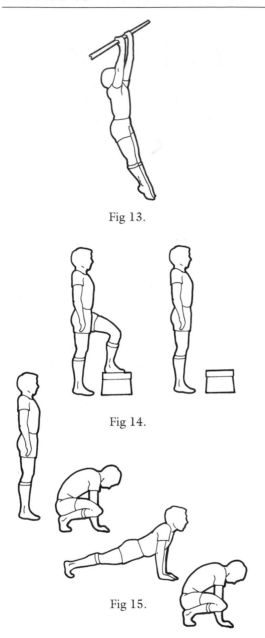

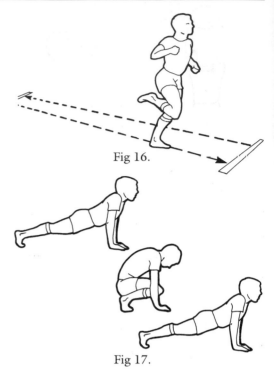

Fig 13.

Fig 16.

Fig 14.

Fig 17.

Fig 15.

9. *Shuttle run (Fig 16)* Sprint continuously between two lines 10 metres apart and touch the line on the floor at each turn.

10. *Squat thrust (Fig 17)* Front support position: jump both feet to crouch position, then jump both feet back to front support. Repeat rhythmically and continuously.

11. *Side bend (Fig 18)* Hold medicine ball above head with straight arms: with a controlled movement bend over on right side, then across to the left: keep arms straight and behind line of the ears.

12. *Skipping (Fig 19)* With suitable rope, maintain continuous, rhythmical skipping.

8. *Burpee (Fig 15)* From standing position crouch to place hands on the floor in front of the feet, jump both feet back to front support position: then jump both feet back to crouch position and stand up. Repeat the complete movement rhythmically and continuously.

Start at any of the twelve stations and continue in order prescribed. The interval of work could be 30 seconds or 60 seconds, with an interval of rest of 30 seconds. Alternatively, a prescribed number of repetitions can be given for each exercise and by increasing

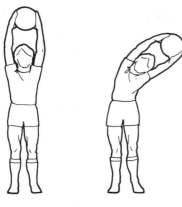 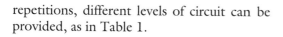 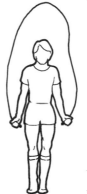 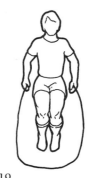

Fig 18.

Fig 19.

repetitions, different levels of circuit can be provided, as in Table 1.

Circuit B – General Fitness Circuit

Circuit B is a second example of a general fitness circuit, but it indicates the possible variation by using partners, and how work on a circuit can be recorded to monitor progress. It also introduces gymnasium equipment into the circuit.

1. *Agility run (Fig 20)* Sprint in between a row of four skittles, to one end and back: alternate with partner.
2. *Bench press (Fig 21)* Both partners lie on back with ends of a gymnasium bench held in front of the chest with arms straight: working together, lower and push up the bench.
3. *Bench crossover jumping (Fig 22)* With feet together, jump diagonally across the bench working from end to end: one partner follows the other.

Table 1 Suggested number of repetitions for each exercise.

		Red	Green	Black
1.	Push-up	5	10	20
2.	Vertical jump	10	20	30
3.	Abdominal curl	12	21	30
4.	Back extension	10	15	20
5.	Astride jumping (over bench)	12	20	30
6.	Pull up	5	10	15
7.	Bench stepping	15	30	40
8.	Burpee	12	20	30
9.	Shuttle run	10	18	26
10.	Squat thrust	12	20	30
11.	Side bend (holding medicine ball)	10	15	20
12.	Skipping	20	30	40

Note: the repetitions are a guide to providing progression as fitness increases. The levels of effort, thus the number of repetitions, should suit the individual.

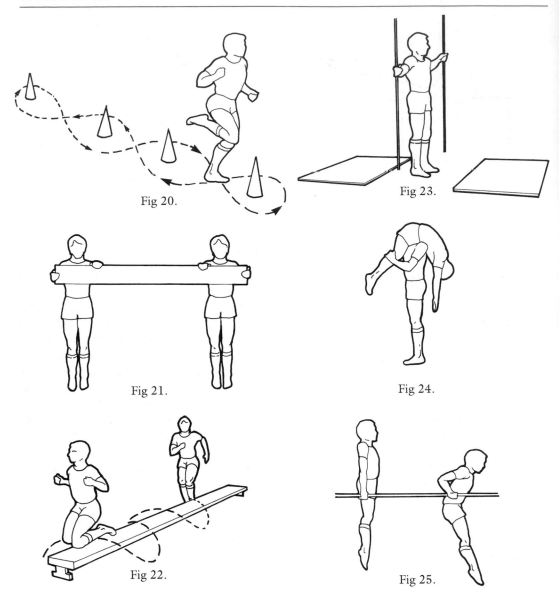

Fig 20.

Fig 21.

Fig 22.

Fig 23.

Fig 24.

Fig 25.

4. *Rope swing (Fig 23)* Each partner stands between two ropes and takes a grip just above shoulder height: two mats are placed either side of the ropes and each partner swings from mat to mat without touching floor in between: both partners working at same time.
5. *Fireman's lift (or Piggy back) (Fig 24)* One partner carries the other partner to a point 10 metres away and then returns: change places.
6. *Dips (Fig 25)* Partners at either end of parallel bars with arms straight positioned above the bars: lower the body so that the elbow joint is at right angles and push back to straight arm position: both partners working at same time.
7. *Back extension (Fig 26)* One partner lies on

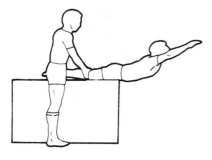

Fig 26.

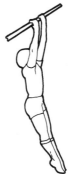

Fig 27.

top of a three-section box with feet along the top surface: the other partner holds the legs down: from flexed position with head on floor, raise the trunk and extend the back: each partner works for half the time.

8. *Pull-up (Fig 27)* Stand below a beam and use undergrasp hold: pull up to touch the beam with chin: the exercise can be made easier by using an inclined pull up position with feet on the floor.

Note – this is an example circuit. Many other exercises can be used, depending on the requirements of the circuit and the availability of equipment. Each repetition is counted and recorded as a team performance (Table 2).

Circuit C – Competitive Circuit

Circuit C introduces a time control by means of putting out and bringing back skittles. It is known as a competitive *circuit*. The number of repetitions are counted and recorded (in a similar way to the method defined for the previous circuit) on all stations except the skittles exercise. The faster the skittles are put out and brought back the shorter the time interval to complete the repetitions on the other exercises. This approach is very suitable to use with younger athletes. The athletes work in pairs. One partner puts out the four skittles as quickly as possible, one at a time on marks set

Exercise	Repetitions		Team Points
	Partner A	Partner B	
Agility Run			
Bench Press			
Bench Crossover Jumping			
Rope Swing			
Fireman's Lift			
Dips			
Back Extension			
Pull-up			
		Total	

Table 2 Record form for Circuit B.

2 metres apart; when this is completed his/her partner sprints out and returns the skittles to the start, one at a time: the interval of work is finished when the last skittle has been returned.

At all other stations, a selection of exercises can be used, again working in pairs and counting repetitions; push-up, abdominal curls, jumping astride a bench, burpee, rope climb, squat thrust and many other similar exercises which allow repetitions to be recorded.

Again, as a team or as individuals, repetitions can be recorded on a form which can provide a rank order amongst a group based on total scores.

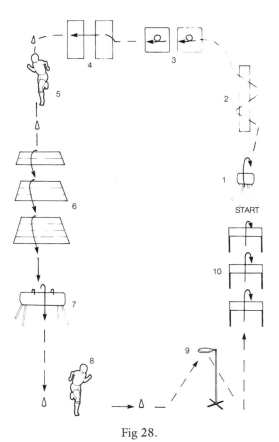

Fig 28.

Circuit D – Continuous Circuit *(Fig 28)*

Circuit D is an example of a circuit using a different method of organization of work. Instead of a set of exercises at each station on a rotation basis, the continuous circuit involves moving around a circuit employing exercises which allow the participants to keep moving forwards. The organization can use partners, with one partner moving around the circuit for a set time interval, say 60 seconds, whilst the other partner rests. The partners then alternate; or instead, one partner completes five circuits and then rests whilst the other partner does the same. In both methods, a decision will have to be made on how many sets to use. The following is a possible plan for a continuous activity circuit.

1. Vault over the buck.
2. Double-footed jumps over a bench, working forwards.
3. Two forward rolls on mats, working forwards.
4. Steeplechase jump: run up to three-section box, jump for second box (three sections) placed a suitable distance away.
5. Sprint 10 metres between two skittles.
6. Continuous run up three boxes (2-section, 3-section and 4-section) placed suitable distances apart.
7. Through vault over the horse.
8. Sprint 10 metres between two skittles.
9. Jump to touch basketball net or backboard.
10. Double footed jumps over three hurdles of suitable height 1 metre apart.

ANAEROBIC CIRCUIT

This approach, using intervals of high level work interspersed with set rest periods, can be used to develop an athlete's anaerobic capacity. The anaerobic fitness circuit outlined

(Fig 39) includes a selection of exercises which can be adapted to the more specific muscular activity of a particular sport, or to concentrate on certain muscle groups. The circuit should be preceded by at least ten minutes warm-up including flexibility work.

Work in pairs; each athlete will work for 30 seconds on each exercise alternating with his/her partner. There will be a one minute rest between each set of exercises. This means that each athlete will rest for one minute and thirty seconds, which gives a work-to-rest ratio of 1:3. The exercises should be done at maximal or near-maximal level and the work/rest intervals tightly controlled.

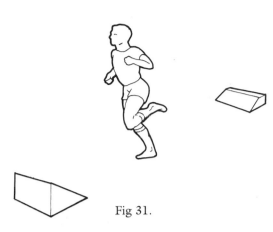

Fig 31.

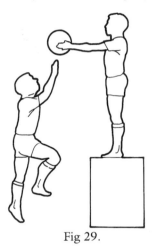

Fig 29.

1. *Box rebound (Fig 29)* Partner A stands on a five-section box holding a ball about half a metre above the reach of partner B; B jumps to take ball, lands, then jumps to return ball to A on the box; work continuously.

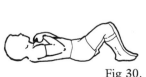

Fig 30.

2. *Abdominal curl (Fig 30)* Lie on back with knees bent and hands across chest; feet should be fixed. Raise trunk and touch both knees with both elbows.

3. *Shuttle run (Fig 31)* Sprint continuously between two inclined turning boards, 10 metres apart.

4. *Inclined pull-up (Fig 32)* Undergrasp on a beam or bar with inclined body position and heels in contact with the floor; pull up to bring chest near to beam.

5. *Bicycle ergometer (Fig 33)* Use a selected load, pedal as fast as possible but keeping contact with the seat throughout the exercise.

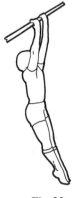

Fig 32.

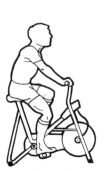

Fig 33.

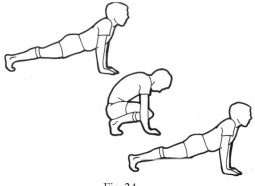

Fig 34.

6. *Squat thrust (Fig 34)* Front support position; jump both feet to crouch position, then jump both feet back to front support.

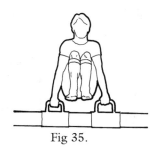

Fig 35.

7. *Beam saddle (Fig 35)* Fix beam at appropriate height; hold handles of beam saddle, jump through saddle with both feet together to land on other side of beam; turn and repeat.

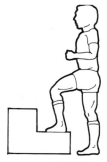

Fig 36

8. *Step up (Fig 36)* Run quickly up benches set in the form of two steps (or suitable staircase); return to starting position and repeat.

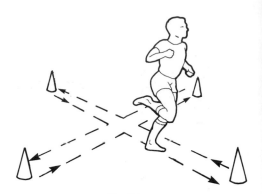

Fig 37.

9. *Star run (Fig 37)* Four skittles are set out at the corners of a square, 5 metres apart. Stand in the middle of the square, sprint to a skittle and return to the middle; repeat this working round the four skittles returning to the middle each time.

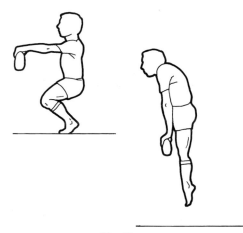

Fig 38.

10. *Beam push-up (Fig 38)* Stand in front of a beam which is set at waist height; hold beam and drop down into squat position; drive up to balance on beam and repeat.

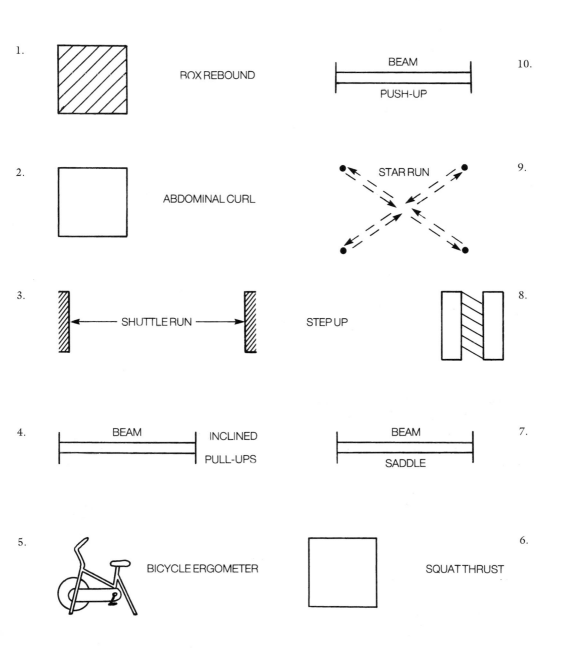

Fig 39 Layout of the anaerobic circuit.

SPORT-SPECIFIC CIRCUIT

All athletes involved in sport require a basic level of general fitness which will include the ability of the cardio-respiratory system to respond to exercise, muscular endurance, flexibility, strength and power, but onto this basis must be built specific fitness which prepares the body to meet the specific demands of a sport.

Circuit training can help to prepare you for your sport by improving basic fitness, but it can be used more specifically to build up muscular endurance in those muscles used primarily in the sport and by having particular and appropriate effects on the cardio-vascular system.

In preparing a sport-specific circuit, certain factors need to be considered:

1. The skills involved in the sport. From an analysis of the muscular actions involved, various exercises and activities will be devised.
2. The cardio-respiratory requirements of the sport. The length of time for each exercise and the length of the recovery period will depend upon this assessment; and these times will depend upon the fitness of the athletes engaged in the circuit.
3. The availability of equipment, the best use of floor space together with the numbers involved in the training.

The following section includes examples of sport specific work. These should provide ideas for the kind of exercise that can be used for individual sports. The circuits can be modified according to particular needs, other exercises can be devised with a little thought, and general fitness exercises can be added to give a fuller programme of work. Intervals of work and rest can be altered to suit different ages and levels of fitness. A points system can be worked into circuits if desired to provide a form of competition between the participants.

Association Football Circuit

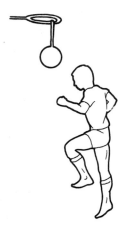

Fig 40.

1. *Sprint and head (Fig 40)* Sprint 10 metres, then jump to head a football suspended from a basketball ring: one partner follows the other.
2. *Throw in (Fig 41)* Throw in using a medicine ball: throw to partner who returns.

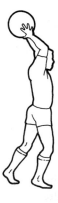

Fig 41.

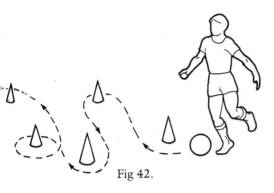

Fig 42.

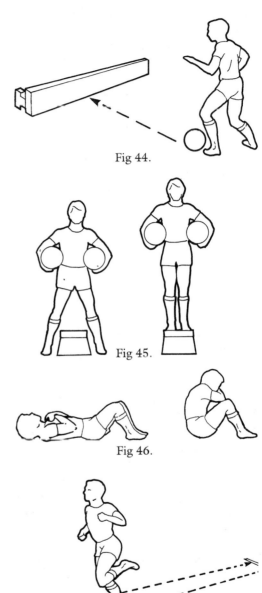

Fig 44.

3. *Dribbling (Fig 42)* Dribbling a football around course marked out with skittles: follow partner.

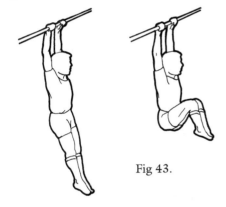

Fig 43.

Fig 45.

Fig 46.

4. *Wallbar knee raise (Fig 43)* Hang from wallbars, raise knees to chest and lower: partners work together.

5. *Dribble and return (Fig 44)* Dribble a football 10 metres, push pass ball against a bench turned on its side, collect pass and return to start line: partners alternate.

6. *Astride jumps (Fig 45)* Astride jumping on and off a bench with a medicine ball under each arm: partners work at either end of bench.

7. *Abdominal curl (Fig 46)* Lie on back with knees bent and hands across chest, curl up and twist touching left knee with right elbow; then repeat touching right knee with left elbow, continue alternating in this way: both partners working.

Fig 47.

8. *Shuttle run (Fig 47)* Sprint out to line 15 metres away and sprint back: alternate with partner.

9. *Back extension (Fig 48)* Partner A lies across top section of a box holding medicine ball; partner B holds his feet: A raises his trunk above the level of the box and then lowers carefully: partners change half way.

10. *Hurdle jump (Fig 49)* Set out four hurdles 50–70cm high, 1 metre apart; double-footed jumps continuously over the four hurdles; turn and repeat: one behind the other.

11. *Straight arm overthrow (Fig 50)* Partners lie on floor a suitable distance apart; from lying position with ball in the hands on the floor,

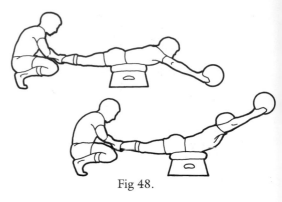

Fig 48.

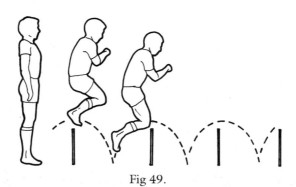

Fig 49.

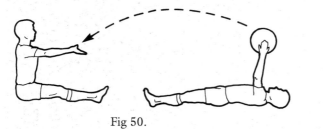

Fig 50.

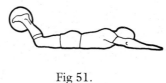

Fig 51.

throw ball to partner keeping upper back on the floor: then sit up to receive ball from partner.

12. *Leg curl (Fig 51)* Prone position on the floor and grip a medicine ball between the feet; raise ball by flexing knees as far as possible: both partners working.

Organization: work in pairs with a suggested work interval of 30 seconds, interval of rest 20 seconds.

Additional exercises for goalkeepers:

1. *High ball (Fig 52)* Partner A stands on a high box holding a ball out with straight arms; partner B runs in from 3 metres, jumps to take the ball, runs to touch a wall 5 metres away, runs back and jumps to return ball to partner A: partners change half way.

2. *Rebound (Fig 53)* Both partners face a wall; Partner A throws ball with overarm action high

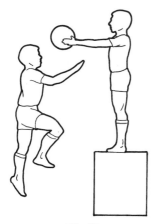

Fig 52.

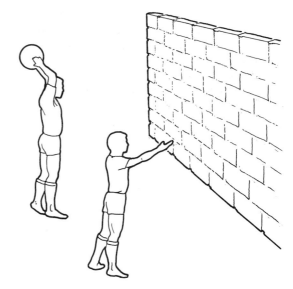

Fig 53.

on to the wall, partner B fields the rebound and then throws for partner A to receive.

3. *Catching (Fig 55)* Partner A lies prone on a mat; partner B throws ball to A so that he has to move quickly in a different direction to catch it; he should catch with both hands and remain on the mat: partners change half way.

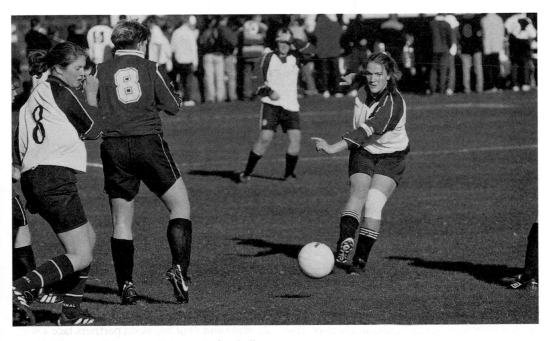

Fig 54. The growing sport of women's football.

39

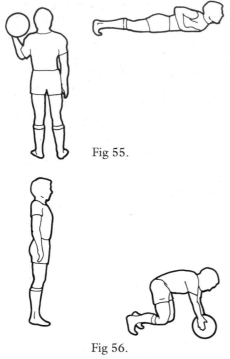

Fig 55.

Fig 56.

5. *Goal-saving (Fig 57)* A suitable mat surface is set out in front of a goal marked on a wall; partner A stands in front of the goal and partner B shoots in different directions by throwing the ball; a number of balls are used in order to keep A continually on the move: partners change half way.

Suggested work interval 60 seconds, with partners changing over half way where indicated.

Basketball Circuit

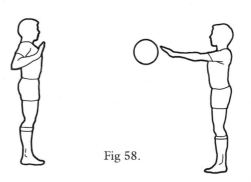

Fig 58.

4. *Diving (Fig 56)* Partner A runs in 10 metres, dives to pick up a ball on a mat, runs to touch wall, runs back to mat, replaces ball, does a forward roll and runs back to start line: partner B starts as soon as the ball has been replaced on the mat.

1. *Chest passing (Fig 58)* Partners stand 5 metres apart and chest pass as quickly as possible.

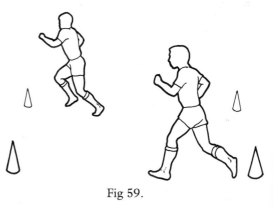

Fig 59.

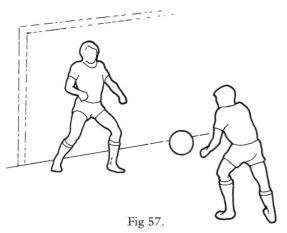

Fig 57.

2. *Running the square (Fig 59)* Four skittles are placed to form a square with sides of about 6 metres; partners run around the square in

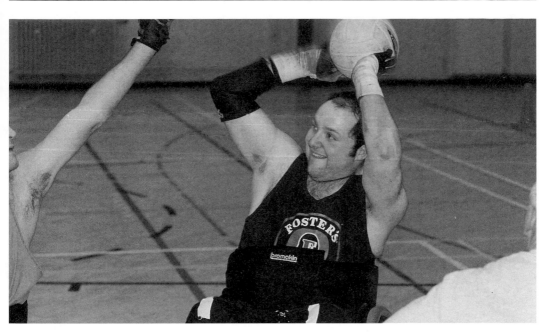

Fig 60 Ready to shoot in basketball.

opposite directions so they have to use peripheral vision to avoid collision.

3. *Box rebound (Fig 61)* Partner A stands on a five-section box holding a ball about half a metre above partner B's reach. B jumps to take ball, lands, then jumps to return ball to A on the box: partners change half way.

4. *Wall-tipping (Fig 62)* Both partners stand facing a wall and tip a ball against the wall, with arms held up, keeping the ball above a line at a height of 3 metres.

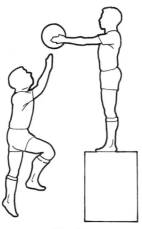

Fig 61.

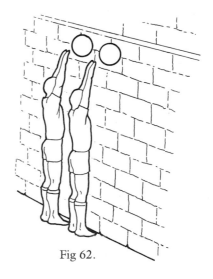

Fig 62.

41

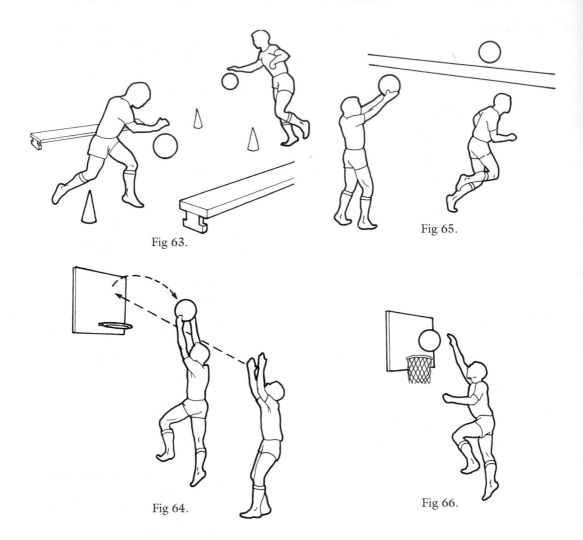

Fig 63.

Fig 65.

Fig 64.

Fig 66.

5. *Dribbling maze (Fig 63)* Benches and skittles are set out to form a maze; partners dribble ball round the maze in opposite directions.

6. *Rebounding (Fig 64)* Partner A throws ball on to backboard; partner B jumps high to take ball on the rebound, arms fully extended; B then throws ball for A to do likewise.

7. *High chest passing (Fig 65)* A beam is set out at 3 metres; both partners working, pass the ball over the beam from a range of 2 metres, then run to a similar point on the other side of the beam to catch the ball after the first bounce: the ball is then passed back again.

8. *Lay-up (Fig 66)* Stand 5 metres away from the basket, dribble the ball in and execute a lay-up shot first from the right, then from the left: keep alternating with one partner following the other.

Work in pairs, with a suggested work interval of 120 seconds. Interval of rest, 20 seconds.

Cricket Circuit

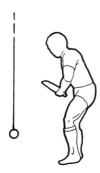

Fig 67.

1. *Batting (Fig 67)* Suspend a ball about 10cm from the floor with some form of cushioning surface (mat positioned vertically) just over 1 metre away from it: partner A drives the ball at the 'mat', and runs forward to a line 4 metres away: he runs back, takes up the correct stance again, and makes another shot. Partner B stops the ball and steadies it for the next shot: partners change half way.

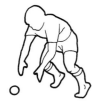

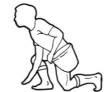

Fig 68.

2. *Fielding (Fig 68)* A basket is placed at each side of the gymnasium/hall; partner A has a container of tennis balls in the centre and gently rolls one at a time midway between the baskets; partner B runs in, picks up the ball, runs and places ball in far basket; he then runs back to pick up the next ball which is then placed in the other basket: partners change half way.

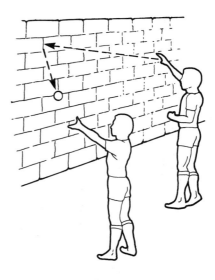

Fig 69.

3. *Catching (Fig 69)* Both partners stand facing a wall at a distance of about 5 metres; partner A throws at a target marked on the wall and partner B catches the rebound: B then throws for A.

4. *Running between wickets (Fig 70)* Mats are placed at each side of the gymnasium/hall about 20 metres apart; each partner runs between mats with a bat in hand, touching the mat at each end.

5. *Wicket-keeping (Fig 71)* Partner A takes up wicket-keeper's squatting position behind a skittle (wicket); partner B throws ball alternately to 'off' side and 'leg' side; A moves to take the ball, always returning to the squatting position: partners change half way.

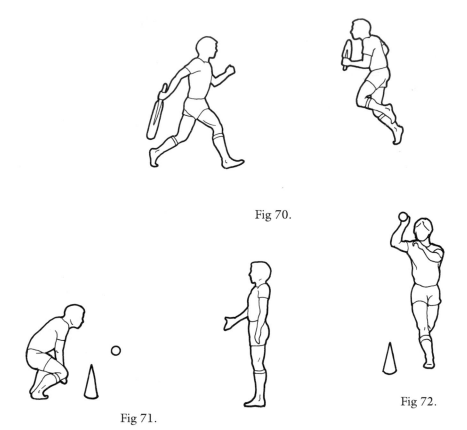

Fig 70.

Fig 71.

Fig 72.

6. *Bowling (Fig 72)* Set up two skittles (wickets) standard distance apart; partner A takes a normal run from one end and bowls for the far target and follows through to cross a line 3 metres in front of the skittle; he then runs back to bowl again; partner B collects the deliveries and feeds A: partners change half way.

7. *Fielding (Fig 73)* Partners stand together on one side of the gymnasium/hall; partner A rolls a ball across the floor, partner B sprints out and picks up the ball and both run to the far side; B then rolls the ball back for A to pick up.

Work in pairs, with a suggested work interval of 120 seconds. Interval of rest, 30 seconds.

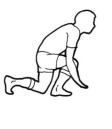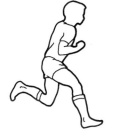

Fig 73.

Gymnastics Circuit

1. *Push-up (Fig 74)* Adopt the front support position. Bend arms so that the chest touches the floor each time; arms must be fully extended on the return, back must be kept straight; height of feet above floor (using bench, wallbars) can be used to increase resistance.

2. *Sargent jump (Fig 75)* From standing position, lower body and execute an explosive vertical jump with half twist to face a wall.

3. *Pull-up (Fig 76)* Stand below a beam and use undergrasp hold; pull up to touch the beam with chin. The exercise can be made easier by using an inclined pull-up position with feet on the floor.

4. *Hopping (Fig 77)* Move forward and back across a distance of 10 metres; use a sequence of hopping on the left foot for one length, on the right foot for the next length, followed by double-footed jumps.

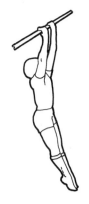

Fig 76.

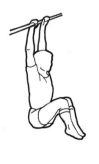

Fig 77.

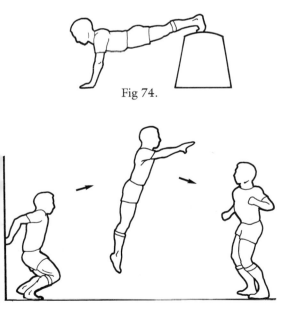

Fig 74.

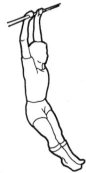

Fig 78.

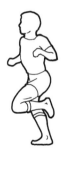

Fig 75.

5. *Leg raise and swing (Fig 78)* Hang from wallbars and lift knees to chest; this can be alternated with legs and trunk swinging sideways with controlled movements.

45

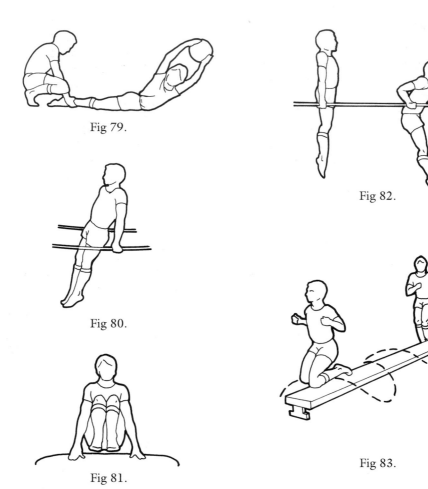

Fig 79.

Fig 80.

Fig 81.

Fig 82.

Fig 83.

6. *Back extension (Fig 79)* Lie on floor with feet fixed (by a partner); raise trunk from floor with twist; repeat to the other side. A medicine ball can be used for added resistance.

7. *Body swing (Fig 80)* Adopt position above parallel bars; swing with straight arms and keep legs and body straight.

8. *Through vault (Fig 81)* Execute a simple through vault over a box; run back and repeat.

9. *Dips (Fig 82)* Adopt position above parallel bars; lower body until elbow joint is at right angles, then press back to straight arm position.

10. *Bench crossover jumping (Fig 83)* Stand to one side of the end of a bench, facing along the length of the bench: jump diagonally across the bench and continue jumping from side to side down the bench; return by repeating the same movements backwards along the bench.

Work as individuals or in pairs, with a suggested work interval of 30 seconds. Suggested interval of rest, 10 seconds. Circuit can be repeated as required after two minutes' rest.

Hockey Circuit

1. *Box jump (Fig 84)* Carrying hockey stick throughout, run 3 metres and jump over three sections of a box; cross line on floor 3 metres from box; back over box and return to line: both partners working.

2. *Ankle running (Fig 85)* Run out to a line 10 metres away and back with hands near to or touching ankles: alternate with partner.

3. *Wall press (Fig 86)* Partner A pushes partner B gently towards a wall from a distance of one metre; B places hands on the wall, bends the arms fully and pushes back vigorously; A catches B and pushes back again: partners change half way.

4. *Control and pass (Fig 87)* Partner A rolls ball to partner B, who stops the ball inside a 1 metre diameter circle using his hockey stick, dribbles round a marker 3 metres away and back to the circle, then push passes ball back to A: partners change half way.

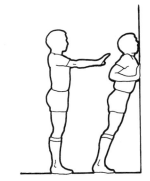

Fig 86.

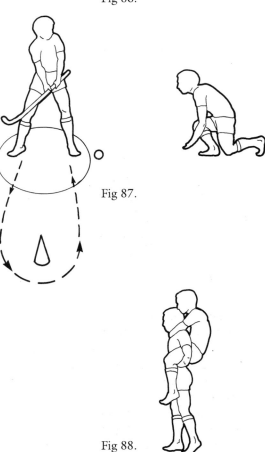

Fig 87.

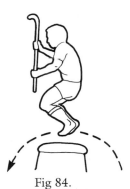

Fig 84.

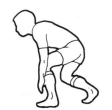

Fig 85.

Fig 88.

5. *Partner carry (Fig 88)* Partner A carries partner B using piggy back or fireman's lift for 10 metres: then change position and return.

47

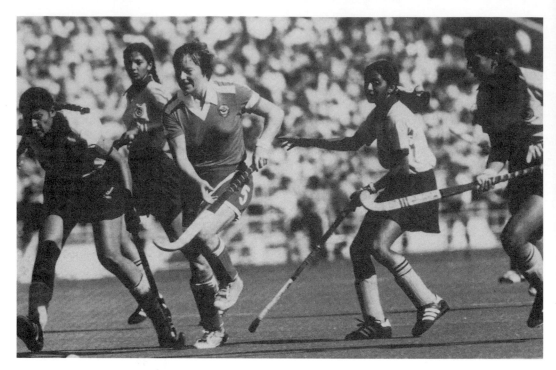

Fig 89 International hockey action.

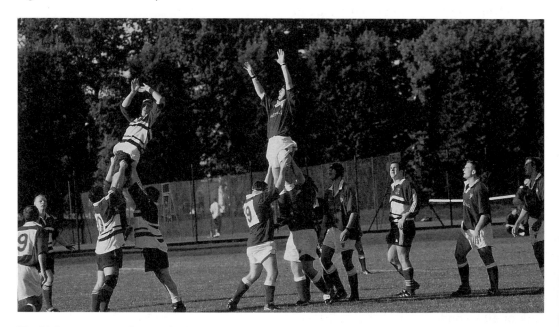

Fig 90 Leg power and upper body strength in a line-out in rugby football.

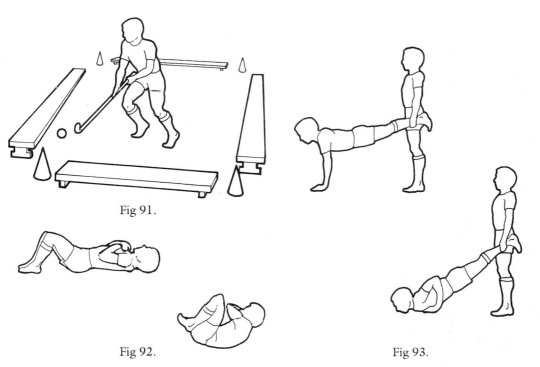

Fig 91.

Fig 92.

Fig 93.

6. *Dribbling maze (Fig 91)* Set out a maze of skittles and benches; partners dribble ball around the maze working in opposite directions.

7. *Knee and chest raise (Fig 92)* Lie on back with knees bent and hands across chest; raise trunk and bring knees to chest at the same time.

8. *Elevated push-up (Fig 93)* Partner A adopts front support position and partner B lifts up his legs into a wheelbarrow hold; A lowers his chest to floor and then presses back: partners change half way.

9. *Depth jump (Fig 94)* Partner A adopts a front support kneeling position; partner B double-footed jumps over A's back, turns and repeats movement: partners change half way.

Work in pairs, with a suggested interval of work of 40 seconds. Interval of rest, 20 seconds.

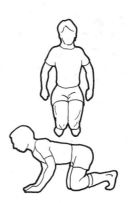

Fig 94.

49

Rowing or Canoeing Circuit

1. *Double-footed jump (Fig 95)* From a squat position, drive forward and upward with feet together to a line 5 or 6 metres away; gently run back and repeat.

2. *Walk-up (Fig 96)* Adopt the front support position and walk up to hands keeping legs straight, then return to front support position: this exercise should be done continuously.

3. *Back extension (Fig 97)* Partner A lies along top section of a box holding a medicine ball with trunk flexed; partner B holds his feet securely; A raises his trunk above level of the box and then lowers carefully; partners change half way.

4. *Vertical jump (Fig 98)* From position of kneeling on one leg with fingers touching floor, jump up and change legs to land in opposite kneeling position.

5. *Wrist roller (Fig 99)* Attach a suitable weight by a length of cord to a bar or section of an oar/paddle; by rotating the bar, roll up and unroll the weight.

6. *Abdominal curl (Fig 100)* Lie on back with knees bent and hands across the chest; curl up and twist, touching left knee with right elbow; then repeat touching right knee with left elbow: continue alternating in this way.

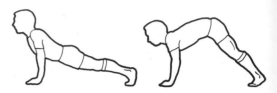

Fig 96.

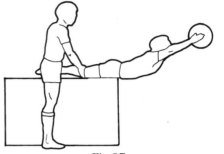

Fig 97.

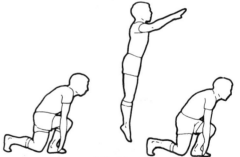

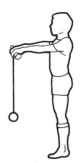

Fig 98.

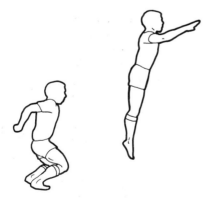

Fig 95.

Fig 99.

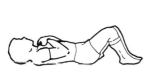

Fig 100.

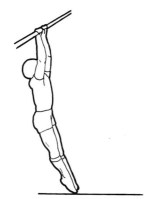

Fig 101.

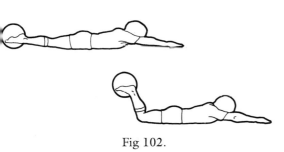

Fig 102.

Rugby Football Circuit

1. *Leg thrust (Fig 103)* Partner A lies on back with legs raised and held out straight; partner B holds on to A's feet and then presses A's knees and hips into full flexion; A then presses and straightens legs against the resistance which B provides: partners change half way.

2. *Scrum-half pass (Fig 104)* Partners stand 3 metres apart; ball is placed on floor by partner A who, after passing to partner B, runs back to a mark 5 metres away and then returns to receive the pass from B, who repeats the same activity.

3. *Mat tackle (Fig 105)* Partner A holds a tackle bag in the middle of an expanse of crash mats; partner B runs from a distance of 5 metres and tackles the bag; A then runs to start line, while B replaces the bag and holds it for A to tackle.

4. *Pick up on the run (Fig 106)* Both partners stand on a line with partner A holding ball; A then rolls ball forward for partner B to run out and pick up; both partners run to an opposite line 10 metres away; B then rolls ball for A to run and pick up.

7. *Horizontal inclined pull-up (Fig 101)* Adopt a horizontal or inclined body position; pull up to bar using an overgrasp grip.

8. *Leg curl (Fig 102)* Prone position on the floor and grip medicine ball between the feet; raise ball by flexing knees as far as possible.

Work individually or in pairs, with a suggested interval of work of 60 seconds. Interval of rest, 15 seconds.

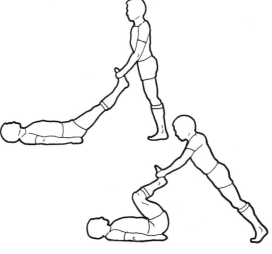

Fig 103.

51

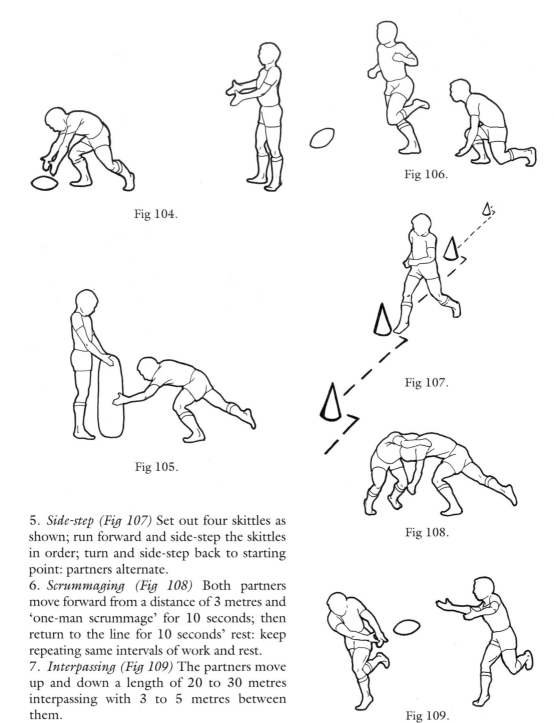

Fig 104.

Fig 105.

Fig 106.

Fig 107.

Fig 108.

Fig 109.

5. *Side-step (Fig 107)* Set out four skittles as shown; run forward and side-step the skittles in order; turn and side-step back to starting point: partners alternate.

6. *Scrummaging (Fig 108)* Both partners move forward from a distance of 3 metres and 'one-man scrummage' for 10 seconds; then return to the line for 10 seconds' rest: keep repeating same intervals of work and rest.

7. *Interpassing (Fig 109)* The partners move up and down a length of 20 to 30 metres interpassing with 3 to 5 metres between them.

8. *Box rebound (Fig 110)* Partner A stands on a five section box holding a ball about half a metre above partner B's reach; B jumps to take ball, lands, then jumps to return ball to A on the box: partners change half way.

9. *Shuttle run (Fig 111)* From a starting line, run to a line 5 metres away and run back, then to a line 10 metres away and back; finally to a line 15 metres away and back: alternate with partner.

Work in pairs, with a suggested interval of work of 60 seconds. Interval of rest, 15 seconds.

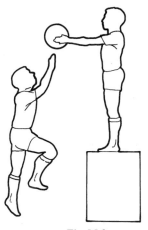

Fig 110.

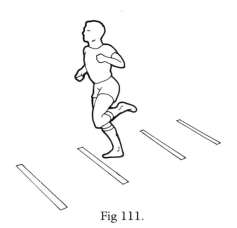

Fig 111.

Skiing Circuit

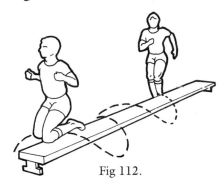

Fig 112.

1. *Bench crossover jumping (Fig 112)* Stand to one side of the end of a bench, facing along the length of the bench; jump diagonally across the bench and continue jumping from side to side down the bench; return by repeating the same movements backwards along the bench. Keep body upright and sway sideways from hips: partners work together one after the other.

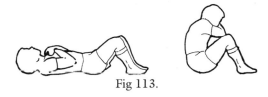

Fig 113.

2. *Abdominal curl (Fig 113)* Lie on back with knees bent and hands across chest; curl up and twist, touching left knee with right elbow, then repeat touching right knee with left elbow; continue alternating in this way: both partners working.

3. *Step-up (Fig 114)* Face and step up onto a high bench; keep on toes and reach as high as possible: both partners working.

4. *Pole planting (Fig 115)* Use two appropriately sized poles with some form of base; hold a pole in each hand (same position as ski-poles) and vault through the poles pushing down hard and backward: both partners working.

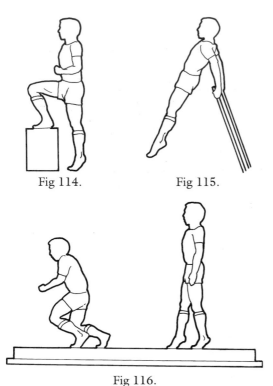

Fig 114.   Fig 115.

Fig 116.

5. *Balance walk (Fig 116)* Balance walk along an upturned bench, lowering body into full squat on each step: alternate with partner.

6. *Straight or bent arm pullover (Fig 117)* Use a suitably weighted bar; lie back on a bench to support head, trunk and hips with feet firmly planted on the floor. Hold bar over the chest with arms straight; gently lower the bar one quarter of a circle so that it is behind the head in line with the top of the bench; after a brief pause return the bar to above the head with straight arms. Breathe in as the bar is taken behind the head, and out as it is returned above the head.

An alternative way of performing this exercise, is to adopt the same position with head as near to end of bench as possible. Then, with elbows at right angles, adopt an overgrasp grip on the bar and carry out a similar exercise with the arms bent; lower the bar behind the head; then return the bar to above the head with bent arms. Breathe in when taking bar back over the head and out as it is taken towards the chest: partners change half way.

7. *Twist and touch (Fig 118)* Stand with the feet parallel; twist to right and try to touch the floor with right hand behind and outside left heel; return to starting position and repeat movement to left; both partners working.

8. *Box rebound (Fig 119)* Partner A stands on a five-section box holding a ball about half a

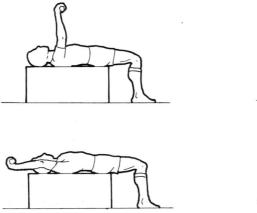
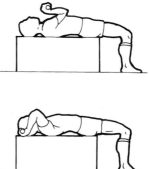

Fig 117 Alternative methods.

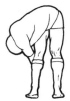

Fig 118.

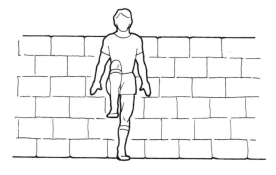

Fig 120.

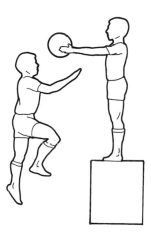

Fig 119.

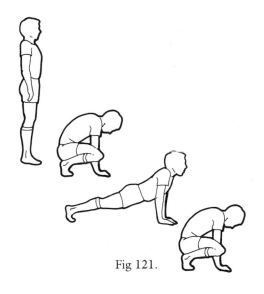

Fig 121.

metre above partner B's reach; B jumps to take ball, lands, then jumps to return ball to A on the box: partners change half way.

9. *Knee raise (Fig 120)* Stand with back to wall and raise alternate knees to chest: both partners working.

10. *Burpee (Fig 121)* From standing position crouch to place hands on the floor in front of the feet, jump both feet back to front support position and stand up; repeat the complete movement rhythmically and continuously: both partners working.

Work in pairs, with a suggested interval of work of 60 seconds. Interval of rest, 20 seconds.

Swimming Circuit

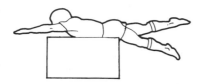

Fig 122.

1. *Flutter kick (Fig 122)* Lie along a box top with body supported to the hips; raise and lower legs using flutter kick action.

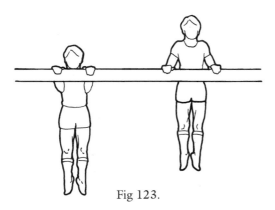

Fig 123.

2. *Muscle up (Fig 123)* Hang from a beam and pull up to chin; then continue by pressing up the beam

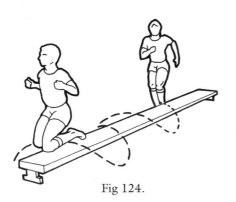

Fig 124.

3. *Bench crossover jumping (Fig 124)* Stand to one side of the end of a bench, facing along the length of the bench; jump diagonally across the bench and continue jumping from side to side down the bench: return by repeating the same movements backwards along the bench.

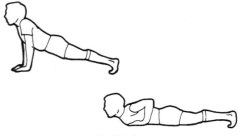

Fig 125.

4. *Abdominal curl (Fig 125)* Lie on back with knees bent and hands across chest; curl up and twist, touching left knee with right elbow; then repeat touching right knee with left elbow; continue alternating in this way: both partners working.

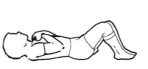

Fig 126.

5. *Push-up (Fig 126)* Adopt the front support position; bend arms so that the chest touches the floor each time; arms must be fully extended on the return, back must be kept straight: progressively work to raise legs.

6. *Shuttle run (Fig 127)* From a starting line, run to a line 5 metres away and run back, then to a line 10 metres away and back; finally to a line 15 metres away and back.

7. *Dips (Fig 128)* Adopt position above parallel bars; lower body until elbow joint is at right angles: then press back to straight arm position.

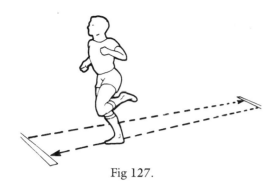

Fig 127.

8. *Leg kick (Fig 129)* Lie prone on high box with legs hanging down over the end; grip box firmly and raise both legs upward extending spine at the same time: keep legs straight and together.

Work individually or in pairs, with a suggested interval of work of 30 seconds. Interval of rest, 15 seconds.

Tennis/Badminton/Squash Circuit

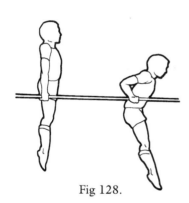

Fig 128.

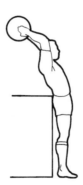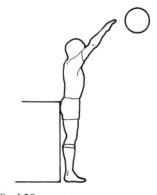

Fig 130.

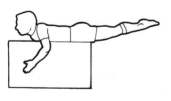

Fig 129.

1. *Medicine ball throw (Fig 130)* Partner A leans back over a buck or box, and throws a medicine ball with an overarm action following through with his body; partner B collects ball and returns to A; partners change half way.

2. *Abdominal curl (Fig 131)* Lie on back with knees bent and hands across chest; curl up and twist, touching left knee with right elbow; then repeat touching right knee with left elbow; continue alternating in this way: both partners working.

3. *Cradle carry (Fig 132)* Partner A carries partner B in cradle position in front of body over a distance of 10 metres; change places and B carries A back to the start.

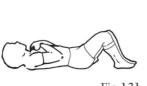

Fig 131.

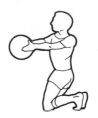

Fig 134.

5. *Trunk rotation (Fig 134)* In the kneeling position, hold a medicine ball out in front of the body with straight arms. Using a controlled movement, move the medicine ball across to one side rotating the trunk as fully as possible; then move the medicine ball right across to the other side always keeping the ball above waist height: both partners working.

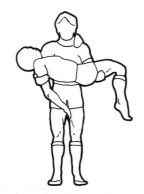

Fig 132.

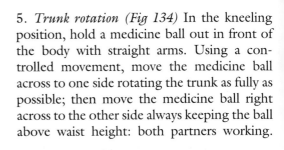

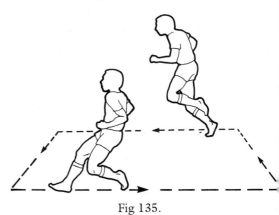

Fig 135.

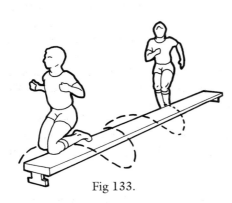

Fig 133.

4. *Bench crossover jumping (Fig 133)* Stand to one side of the end of a bench, facing along the length of the bench; jump diagonally across the bench and continue jumping from side to side down the bench; turn and repeat in the other direction: partners work together one after the other.

6. *Square running (Fig 135)* Use half a tennis court or similar markings. Start at one corner and run forwards to the end of that side, then run sideways across court, still facing the same way; then backwards along the next side, and then sideways to return to the starting point; partners alternate with A resting while B is running one square: then change.

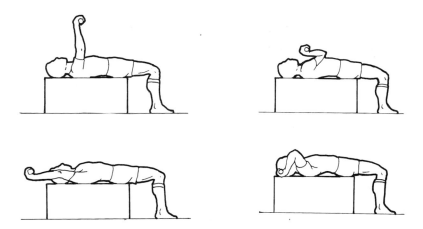

Fig 136 Alternative methods

7. Straight or bent arm pullover (Fig 136) Use a suitably weighted bar; lie back on a bench to support head, trunk and hips with feet firmly planted on the floor. Hold bar over the chest with arms straight; gently lower the bar one quarter of a circle so that it is behind the head in line with the top of the bench; after a brief pause return the bar to above the head with straight arms. Breathe in as the bar is taken behind the head and out as it is returned above the head.

An alternative way of performing this exercise, is to adopt the same position with head as near to end of bench as possible. Then, with elbows at right angles, adopt an overgrasp grip on the bar and carry out a similar exercise with the arms bent; lower the bar behind the head; then return the bar to above the head with bent arms. Breathe in when taking bar back over the head and out as it is taken towards the chest: partners change half way.

8. Kangaroo jump (Fig 137) From standing position explosively bring both knees up to the chest and heels to the seat: both partners working.

Organization: work in pairs, with a suggested work interval of 120 seconds. Interval of rest, 30 seconds.

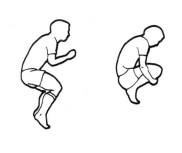

Fig 137.

59

CHAPTER 4
Flexibility

Flexibility is possibly the most neglected and undervalued component of physical fitness, particularly by male athletes. A lack of flexibility, not uncommon in males, can be a cause of poor performance and inefficient technique, as well as a possible underlying cause for many of the strain and tear type muscle injuries found in sport. Poor flexibility can hinder speed and endurance qualities, for the muscle may have to work harder to overcome resistance, and by increasing the possible range of movement in shoulder, hip and ankle joints, for example, greater speed and agility may be achieved as well as saving energy.

But it is important to stress again the need for a balanced approach to fitness training, and to appreciate how the various components of fitness are inter-related. It is a mistake to consider one component, i.e. flexibility or strength, in isolation. As an example, the amount of stretch and thus increased flexibility achieved will not be of benefit unless it is accompanied by an increase in muscle strength. Conversely, many athletes wishing to improve their performance set gains in strength against losses in flexibility. Programmes in strength training may, in fact, limit possible increases in range of movement, or even decrease this quality, bringing about a deterioration in other areas of training. A strength programme (say) using weight training need not result in muscle boundedness or diminished range of movement, if the strength work is compensated with adequate flexibility exercises to provide a balanced approach and subsequent development.

Probably the best argument for increased flexibility is that it will facilitate maximal exploitation of the strengths and abilities of the athlete and, if flexibility is developed to provide for a greater range of movement than is actually required in performance, this can be an effective means of injury prevention.

Regular flexibility training can increase relaxation in the muscles and there is some evidence to show that stretching exercises can help to ease muscular soreness which follows a hard training session or a competition.

FLEXIBILITY TRAINING

It is helpful to understand the nature and structure of a flexibility training programme and particularly to distinguish between a flexibility programme that attempts to increase range of movements in certain joints over a period of time, and flexibility exercises which are included within warm-up and cool-down routines to help with preparing the body for work and with the recovery process after a session or competition.

Stretching exercises and drills have been devised and developed to increase the range of movement in various joints and basically include stretching the muscle beyond its habitual length.

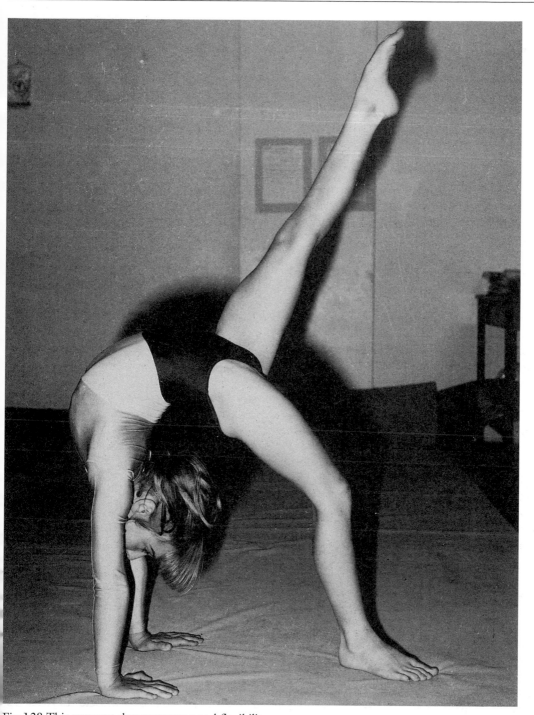

Fig 138 This gymnast demonstrates good flexibility.

Types of Stretching

Stretching involves the lengthening or extending of muscle; there are four basic stretching techniques: ballistic, dynamic, static and proprioceptive. Ballistic, dynamic and static techniques may be done actively. Static and proprioceptive techniques can be done passively.

Active Stretching

Active stretching involves the athlete working alone on flexibility exercises and supplies the force of the stretch. The extra range of movement is achieved by a more complete degree of relaxation in the muscles being stretched, by applying force from the contraction of other muscles and movement of body parts.

Passive Stretching

In passive stretching, the athlete remains relaxed and makes no contribution to the movement of the limb or body part. This is done by an external force, usually another person, a sensible partner. Passive stretching with a partner sensibly applying the force can be valuable because it merely requires relaxation of the muscles under pressure, and with good communication between partners an effective stretch can be achieved.

Ballistic Stretching

Ballistic stretching involves a bouncing or jerking motion with the aim of gaining momentum in the body parts in order to reach further. Its momentum takes the moving limb or part of the body to its limits, including exercises of the 'flinging and swinging' type, the 'bouncing and bobbing' movements. This type of exercise is probably of value for maintaining a range of movement, but it is unlikely to increase the range, because unconsciously one uses only sufficient momentum to take the limb, and the muscles involved, to their present habitual length.

With this method there could be muscle strain, and possibly physical damage due to microscopic tearing of muscle fibres. This tearing can lead to the formation of scar tissue with gradual loss of elasticity. The quick, repetitive bouncing actions will initiate a stretch reflex permitting only a momentary lengthening of the muscle. In addition it is possible that these exercises can produce muscle soreness and even losses in resilience and elasticity.

Dynamic Stretching

Dynamic stretching is similar to ballistic stretching in that it utilizes movement, but the essential difference between ballistic and dynamic stretching is that dynamic does not end the movement with a bouncy or jerky movement. Dynamic stretching can improve flexibility and has distinct value, particularly during a warm-up, as the muscle is stretched at certain velocities and certain movement patterns, and sport-specific actions can be used. In the context of warm-up and cooldown, a combination of dynamic and static stretching would seem a sound approach.

Static Stretching

Static stretching involves slow, sustained exercise that places a muscle in a lengthened position and holds the position for 8 to 30 seconds. Static stretching is the safest method; it is easy to learn; and it has proved to be effective. It includes passive relaxation as the muscle is lengthened. There is less likelihood of injury; it is relaxing; and it can help to relieve muscle soreness. It does not elicit the stretch reflex of the stretched muscle and is more in harmony with one of the main resisters to stretching, the connective tissue which responds better to slow sustained stretches.

Proprioceptive Neuromuscular Facilitation

PNF was originally designed and developed as a rehabilitation procedure and is still used in that context. If used sensibly and carefully it can improve range of movement. A PNF stretch combines alternating contraction and relaxation of prime mover and antagonist muscles which causes neural responses in the muscle that inhibit the contraction of that muscle being stretched. This procedure results in a decrease in resistance and thus an increased range of movement when stretching the muscle. PNF techniques usually require a partner who should be experienced in these techniques for the exercises to be safe and effective.

Approach to Flexibility Exercises

The athlete needs to appreciate that certain dangers exist if flexibility exercises are performed incorrectly through ignorance of or disregarding of the basic guidelines.

1. Do not begin flexibility work until the muscles are thoroughly warmed up. They will be more pliable when they are warm and receiving a good supply of blood. Cold muscles tend to resist stretching, so that any stretching which occurs will be directed to the tendons and ligaments. A convenient way to warm up is jogging, followed by light exercises. It is sensible to wear some warm clothing during flexibility, so that the increased body temperature is maintained.
2. The warm-up should be followed with 10 to 15 seconds of *easy* stretching for *each* exercise.

This should cause mild tension in the muscle (or muscles), which should then be relaxed so that the feeling of tension disappears. This preliminary easy stretching helps to reduce any tightness in the muscles and prepares them for the serious flexibility work to follow.

3. When involved in full flexibility work ease into the stretch position to a point where tension is felt but it is comfortable. Do not strain; it should not be painful. (Overdoing the stretching and feeling pain has discouraged athletes from flexibility work.) When the muscles are under stretch, the athlete should experience 'mild discomfort' – nothing more.
4. The stretched position should be held from 10 to 20 seconds and, whilst holding this position, two factors are important. Firstly, as the feeling of stretching decreases, stretch a little further, but ensure that it still feels comfortable and do not bounce in the end position, because of the strain on the muscles being stretched. Secondly, attempt to stretch so that the pull is felt in the bulky central part of the muscle (the 'belly'). If the pulling sensation is felt near the joints, then stress is being put on the tendons and ligaments.
5. It is important to be relaxed during flexibility exercises. Do not hold your breath – breathe calmly and rhythmically during the exercises.
6. It has already been recommended that flexibility work should be included as part of the warm-up to help in preparing the muscles for subsequent exertion and lessen the chances of muscular injury. This would normally be a short session of exercises. The ideal siting for the more serious programme of flexibility exercises would be in the latter part of, or after, a particular training session when the body and muscles are thoroughly warm as a result of the work-out.
7. Frequency of flexibility sessions would depend upon time available and how rapidly

results are required. It may be a priority with certain individuals, and certain sports do demand a high degree of flexibility. The rate of improvement is largely dictated by the amount of work done. Three sessions per week, alternated with other forms of training, would be a typical schedule, but one or two sessions per day should effect quite a rapid improvement.

The following section gives a number of flexibility exercises. The series outlined is designed for sports in general. It is interesting and desirable to devise many similar exercises so that a teacher, coach or athlete has a large and varied programme to select from.

These suggestions can be added to or varied, depending on the athlete's individual strengths and weaknesses and the specific requirements of the sport. Any programme should take a minimum of 10 minutes and, as a guide, up to 30 minutes, but this can vary. The important point is to take your time, to enjoy the exercises and stay relaxed, rather than rushing through the programme just to complete it.

Flexibility Exercises – Active Movements

Look Right and Left (Fig 139)

Starting position: Sit or stand in a position that is comfortable.
Movement Turn head to left and right and hold for 10 seconds.

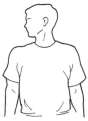

Fig 139.

Repetitions Ten times alternating each direction.

Flexion and Extension (Fig 140)

Starting position Sit or stand in a position that is comfortable.
Movement Flex neck forward by tucking chin in toward the chest; hold for 10 seconds. Extend backward by trying to touch the head to the trapezius; hold for 10 seconds.

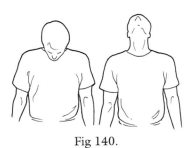

Fig 140.

Shoulders and Chest (Fig 141)

Starting position Stand legs apart; put the elbows behind the head.
Movement Bend sideways at the waist and try to pull the elbows down; keep the arms behind the head.
Time Ten seconds each side.

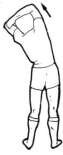

Fig 141.

Arms, Shoulders and Chest (Fig 142)

Starting position Stand legs apart, arms extended overhead and palms together.

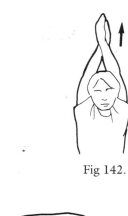

Fig 142.

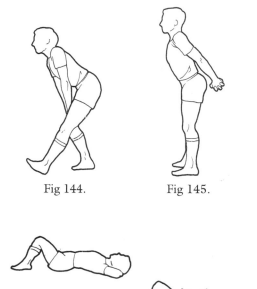

Fig 144.   Fig 145.

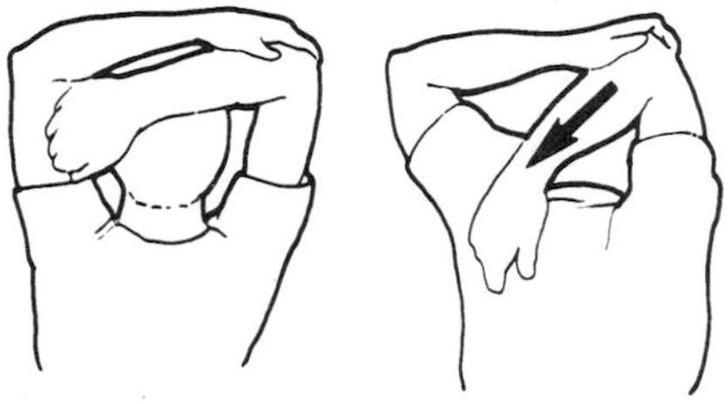

Fig 143.

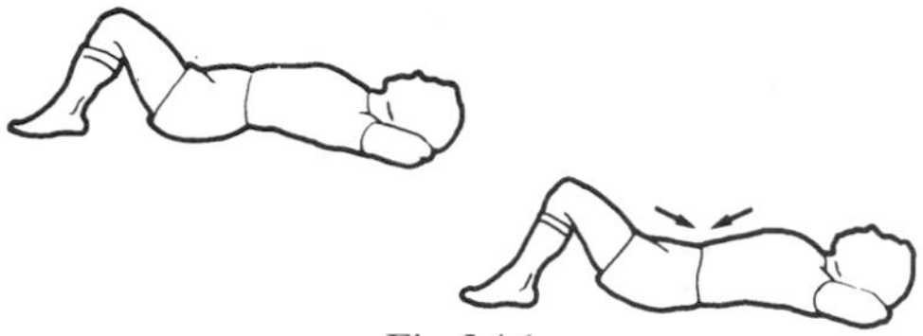

Fig 146.

Movement Stretch arms upward and slightly backward; breathe in while stretching upward.
Time 10 seconds.

Arms and Shoulders (Fig 143)

Starting position Sit or stand legs apart; with arms overhead, hold the elbow of one arm with the hand of the other arm.
Movement Gently pull the elbow behind the head.
Time 10 seconds each arm.

Hamstrings (Fig 144)

Starting position In standing position, place one leg (the leg to be stretched) slightly in front of the other leg. Bend the back leg keeping the back straight and using the hands on the back leg to support the spine. Keep the front leg straight, the head up and prevent the back from curving over.
Movement Press forward until you feel a mild tension.
Time 10 seconds each leg.

Straight Arms behind Back (Fig 145)

Starting position Standing, place both arms behind back. Interlock fingers with palms fac ing each other. Straighten arms fully. Keep head upright and neck relaxed.
Movement Slowly raise the straight arms.
Time Hold for 10 to 15 seconds.

Lower Back (Fig 146)

Starting position Lie on your back with fingers interlaced behind the head and elbows touch-ing the floor: bend the knees. Feet should be shoulder width apart.
Movement Tighten the gluteals (buttocks) and abdominal muscles simultaneously, so that the lower back is flat against the floor.
Time Hold tension for 10 seconds, then relax: repeat three times.

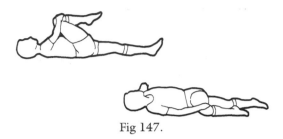

Fig 147.

Time Hold for 10 seconds, then relax.
Second Movement Now turn to face the foot and bend forward in that direction. Try to grasp the ankle.
Time Hold for 10 seconds, then repeat with other leg.
Note This second exercise will also stretch the outer shoulder and chest.

Gluteals (Buttocks) and Hips (Fig 147)

Starting position Lie flat on your back, legs out straight; keep the lower back flat.
First Movement Keeping left leg straight and *flat* to the floor, bend the right leg and grasp below the knee with interlaced fingers; pull right thigh to chest.
Time Hold for 10 seconds and repeat sequence with other leg.
Second Movement Bend the left leg, and with the right hand, pull that bent leg up and over the other straight leg; look to the left shoulder and down the left arm which is extended to the side; keep shoulders flat on the floor and pull the bent leg towards the floor.
Time Hold for 10 seconds and repeat sequence with other leg.

Groin, Hips and Inner Thighs (Fig 148)

Starting position Sit up with the legs spread as wide as they will go, knees locked.
First Movement Slowly bend forward from the hips, keeping quadriceps (top of thighs) relaxed. Try to keep the hips from rolling backward; use the hands out in front for support.

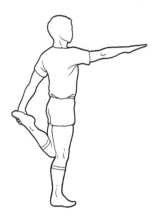

Fig 149.

Quadriceps (Fig 149)

Starting position Stand holding on to something for balance. Flex one knee and raise your heel to the buttocks.
Movement Slightly flex your supporting leg and grasp your raised foot with one hand; slowly pull your heel toward your buttocks without overcompressing the knee.

Groin (Fig 150)

Starting position Sit and put the soles of the feet flat together; hold on to the toes.

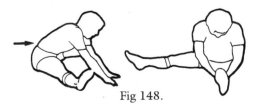

Fig 148.

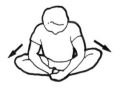

Fig 150.

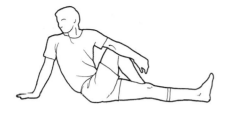

Fig 151.

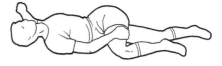

Fig 152.

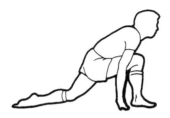

Fig 153.

Movement Gently pull forward, bending from the hips; squeeze knees down with elbows. *Time* 10 seconds.

Spinal Twist (Fig 151)

Starting position Sitting with legs straight and upper body nearly vertical, place right foot on left side of left knee. Place back of left elbow on right side of right knee, which is now bent. Place right palm on floor 30–40cm behind hips.
Movement Push right knee to the left with the left elbow while turning shoulders and head to the right as far as possible. Try to look back.
Time Hold for 10 seconds. Repeat with left leg.

Lower Spinal Twist (Fig 152)

Starting position Lie on your back with your legs extended and your shoulders flat to the floor.
Movement Flex one knee, raise it to your chest, and grasp it with the opposite hand; pull your knee across your body to the floor, keeping your elbows, head and shoulders flat on the floor. This can also be done with the leg straight.

Hips and Quadriceps (Fig 153)

Starting position Place the right foot flat in front; move the right foot forward until the knee is directly over the ankle and the left knee is touching the floor behind, left foot extended.
Movement Lower the hips downward keeping the hips square to the front; use the hands for balance. Check that both feet are in line and not turned out.
Time 10 seconds each leg.
Note To increase the stretch, straighten the back leg and gently lean the trunk up and back. You can push with the arms by placing the hand on the bent knee.

Gastrocnemius and Soleus (Calf) (Fig 154)

Starting position Stand close to and lean on a solid wall (or similar) or partner supporting the body weight on the arms; bend one leg and place the foot in front, with the other leg straight behind.
First Movement Slowly move the hips forward keeping the back flat. Keep the heel of

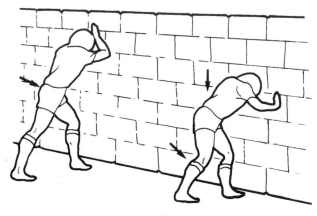

Fig 154.

the straight leg firmly on the floor with the toes pointing straight ahead.

Time Hold for 10 seconds: repeat with other leg.

Second Movement To stretch the lower calf, lower the hips downward as the knees are slightly bending; again, keep the heel down.

Time Hold for 10 seconds, then repeat with other leg.

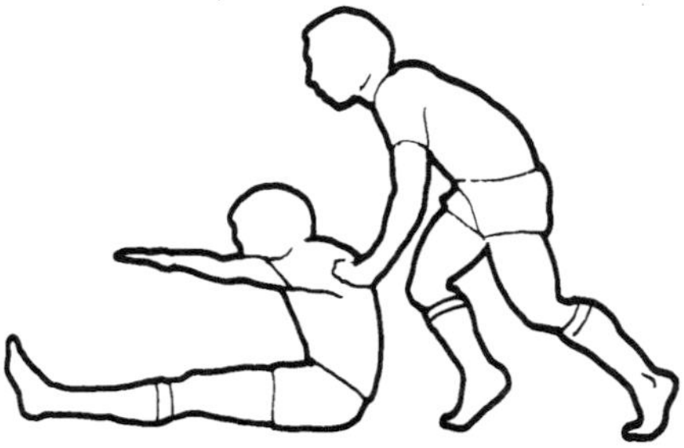

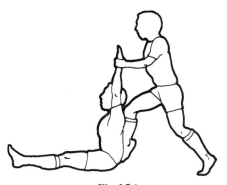

Fig 155.

Flexibility Exercises – Passive Movements

Sitting Press (Fig 155)

A sits on the floor with legs straight; B stands behind, puts hands on A's shoulder blades and presses carefully.

Shoulder Stretch (Fig 156)

A sits on floor with legs straight and arms above the head; B puts the knee against A's back and pulls back A's arms carefully.

Fig 156.

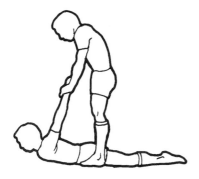

Fig 157.

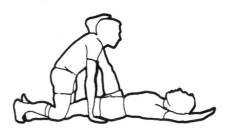

Fig 159.

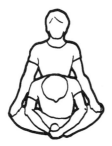

Fig 158.

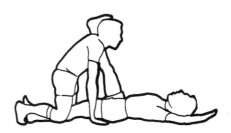

Fig 160.

Lying Shoulder Stretch (Fig 157)

A lies on the floor face downward with arms out to the side; B stands astride A, takes hold of A's arms and pulls them carefully upward.

Butterfly (Groin) (Fig 158)

From a sitting position, A puts the soles of his or her feet together and pulls the heels in as far as possible; he/she relaxes completely and bends at the waist, while B kneels behind and presses his/her chest carefully on A's back, pressing A's knees towards the floor with his/her hands.

Hamstring Stretch (Fig 159)

A lies supine while B lifts one of A's legs with the knee extended, kneeling lightly on the other leg to keep it stabilized. B leans against the raised leg, stretching it carefully for 10 to 15 seconds.

Trunk Rotation (Fig 160)

A lies supine, whilst B moves A's legs across A's body, keeping A's hip flexed and knee extended until A's foot touches the floor. B then applies downward pressure carefully to A's leg and opposite shoulder for 10 to 15 seconds.

69

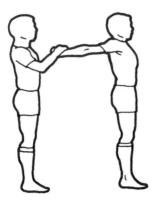

Fig 161.

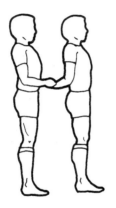

Fig 162.

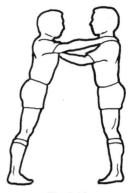

Fig 163.

Shoulder Stretch (External Rotation) (Fig 162)

A stands with upper arms against body, elbows flexed 90 degrees, forearms parallel to the floor and thumbs pointing up. B stands behind, reaches over A's forearms, grasps the hands and pulls the forearms back for 10 seconds, externally rotating A's shoulders.

Calf Stretch (Fig 163)

A stands in front of B with feet together, and leans against B's shoulders keeping feet on the floor. After an initial stretch, A steps further away from B and repeats the stretch, keeping his body rigid and heels close to the floor for 10 seconds.

Shoulder Stretch (Horizontal Abduction) (Fig 161)

A stands with arms raised to the sides parallel with the floor, with thumbs pointing up, B stands behind, reaches under A's arms, grasps A's thumbs and pulls A's arms straight back, slowly and gently. A must relax their arms, stand up straight and keep head up. B pulls A's arms back until mild discomfort is felt; hold for 7 to 10 seconds.

CHAPTER 5
Strength

MUSCULAR CONTRACTION

The development of muscular strength involves a muscle, or group of muscles, exerting a force whilst contracting against a resistance. This contraction involves an increase in muscular tension. There are two general categories of muscle contraction.

1. *Isotonic:* When the muscle contracts, shortening or lengthening occurs during the contraction, with associated movement of body parts.
2. *Isometric:* In performing work, the muscular contraction does not result in movement about the joint axis, but tension is developed.

Isotonic (equal tension) can be further classified into either *concentric* or *eccentric* contractions. In concentric contractions, the muscle actively shortens and thickens with the two end attachments of the muscle, called the points of origin and insertion, moving closer together and the angle at the joint decreasing. A simple example of this would be having your arms outstretched and then flexing the elbow to raise your body towards a bar. The elbow flexor muscles would be contracting concentrically and shortening as the movement took place.

Eccentric contraction occurs when the points of origin and insertion of the muscle are drawn further apart under control. In this case, the muscle will be lengthening and becoming thinner, but it means, of course, that it is returning to its normal resting (habitual) length. An example of eccentric muscle contraction would be lowering slowly down from a previously held undergrasp pull-up position on a bar or beam.

The isometric (equal length) category of muscle contraction is associated with *static* contraction. As the name implies, the length of the muscle remains the same and there is no appreciable joint movement, but tension is developed in the muscle. An example of a static contraction would be a pull-up to a bar or beam and hold a fixed position for a period of time as in the lateral hang.

This brief outline of muscular contraction provides the basis for the development of strength training methods.

TRAINING METHODS

Within the isotonic category the following methods can be identified:

1. Constant resistance.
2. Variable resistance.
3. Accommodating resistance.

Each of these training methods, while isotonic in nature, imposes a different kind of resistance on the working muscle.

Constant Resistance

This is the most widely used method which involves weight training of different types. It can easily be related to the ranges of movement employed in most sports. The constant resistance method of training involves using a constant weight as the muscle contracts, whether it be body weight, barbell or some other form of resistance. Weight training using free weights is an example of this method. Although the resistance remains constant, there is considerable variation in muscle tension during an isotonic contraction, due to continually changing angles at which the muscles apply the force, and alterations in certain biochemical factors. During any particular lift there will be a weak point which represents the weakest joint position in the total range of movement. It is at this point that the muscle will have to do most work. Other parts of the full range of movement will be relatively easier.

Variable Resistance

This method, which is a more recent strength training facility, changes the resistance load on the working muscle group in order to maintain the same relative degree of muscular tension throughout the full range of movement. The reason for this adaptation in resistance is to accommodate the biochemical (leverage) changes which occur during the actual exercise cycle. Some training machines incorporate a design which provides variable resistance throughout the full range of movement. This means that the resistance is automatically increased at those points where the muscles can operate most efficiently and apply greater force, and decreased where the muscles have to apply force from a biomechanically weaker position. It is suggested that, as the resistance is more uniform over the entire range of movement, there should be a greater training effect.

Accommodating Resistance

This method is similar to variable resistance, in that resistance changes take place through the range of movement by controlling the velocity of the contracting muscle. Isokinetic machines, as they are often called, provide a resistance which varies automatically in such a way that it is equal and opposite to the applied muscular force. As the resistance exactly counteracts the applied force, the speed of the muscle contraction is controlled and regulated. A further feature is that a limb velocity which approximates to that used in a sport, for example the arms during front crawl in swimming, can be pre-set to allow the athlete to exert maximum force throughout the entire range of movement on each repetition. There is also accommodating resistance or adjustment to the athlete's varied strength quality at different positions throughout the range of movement.

Static Resistance

Within the isometric category, there is the static resistance training. In this method, muscular force is exerted against a relatively immovable resistance so there is no noticeable limb movement. It is suggested that the approach should involve building tension statically at about two-thirds of maximum effort for 5 to 10 seconds. Strength gains in isometric work will relate directly to the specific angle of the joint at which the training takes place. But if increased strength is required throughout the range, exercises should be performed at a number of joint angles within the range of movement. For this reason, isometric training does have limitations in providing strength increases for athletic performance, but it can provide variety and add to the effects of the more wide-ranging isotonic training methods.

Training Effect

When subjected to the particular kinds of stress outlined, certain adaptations take place within the muscles being worked. The adaptations can be simply outlined as *myogenic* and *neurogenic*. The myogenic adaptations are the muscle fibres responding by increasing their size giving an increase in muscular mass, termed *muscle hypertrophy*. This adaptation will be specific to the nature and intensity of the strength training. There will also be neurogenic improvements, in that the fibres will be more responsive to impulses coming from the central nervous system, the recruitment of the units of fibres within the muscle will be more efficient, and generally the nervous control and response will be better co-ordinated.

There is also research which shows that there is increased thickness and strength of tendons, ligaments and other connective tissue as a result of strength training. Also there is shown to be an increase in the amount of calcium phosphate and calcium carbonate, which increases the strength of the bones. So it appears that a well-structured and appropriate strength training programme develops a number of tissues in the body in addition to muscle development.

APPROACH TO STRENGTH TRAINING

The following provides guidelines for strength training.

You must decide exactly what you are trying to achieve in terms of the nature of the strength required. Everyone should start by developing general strength, but then the programme will be dependent on your sport.

You must relate the programme to the sport or activity in which you perform. After the initial development of general strength, for instance, a rugby football prop-forward would particularly include work on the upper body, arms and shoulders, whereas a volleyball player would want to develop explosive leg power.

You must analyse carefully the muscle groups involved and select the exercises appropriately.

You should be aware of the range and variety of weight training methods. Those athletes who intend to use machines or free weights should seek the help and guidance of a qualified instructor or teacher, or attend a course so that their early experiences of weight training are based on sound and safe principles and techniques, with good supervision in the introductory stages.

You should follow a planned written schedule and calendar of work with regular evaluation of progress. Where possible, training should be recorded on a weight training record card (*Table 3*).

Repetitions The number of times an exercise is performed without stopping.

Sets A specified number of repetitions comprises one set. Three sets of ten repetitions will be written 3×10.

Resistances The load which the muscle (or group of muscles) is required to move. If the resistance is in the form of a measured weight, it will be given in kilograms.

Repetition Maximum The maximum number of times a specified load can be lifted. 10RM is a load that can be lifted just ten times.

If any muscle is to become stronger, it must be put in a state of *overload*. This is done by selecting resistances heavy enough to cause the muscles to work to a certain capacity, and then progressively increase the resistances as the muscle becomes stronger. This is a fundamental principle of a progressive resistance training programme.

Table 3 Weight training record card.

Name				Personal Weight			Sport/Position	

PHASE OF TRAINING

Duration of Training   From: To:

Date:							
Exercise				REPETITION MAXIMUM			
Sets							
Reps							
Kg							
Exercise				REPETITION MAXIMUM			
Sets							
Reps							
Kg							
Exercise				REPETITION MAXIMUM			
Sets							
Reps							
Kg							

At the same time, do not adopt a vague approach to any form of exercising. The exercise prescription should be given bearing in mind the physiological adaptations which result from that exercise. As a general idea, exercises that involve high repetitions and low resistances should improve the endurance qualities of the muscle, whereas low repetitions and high resistances should bring increases in strength. So think in terms of a continuum:

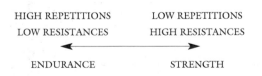

HIGH REPETITIONS   LOW REPETITIONS
LOW RESISTANCES   HIGH RESISTANCES

ENDURANCE   STRENGTH

This is to emphasize that muscular strength and muscular endurance are not separate qualities, but are linked in the way shown and muscle will adapt depending on the training ratio between repetitions and resistances. Absolute muscular strength is at one end of the continuum and absolute endurance at the other. Absolute strength is the maximum force which a muscle can exert against a resistance, the ability to perform one maximal effort or 1RM. Absolute endurance is the maximum capacity of the muscle for continuous performance of localized activity. As a rule, low repetition (3–8 reps) and high resistance work (85–95 per cent of 1RM) is required to produce increases in absolute strength, whereas high repetitions (20–100 reps), low resistance (40–80 per cent of 1RM) work produces increases in muscular endurance.

Power work involves 4–12 reps at maximal speed against a resistance of 60–80 per cent of 1RM.

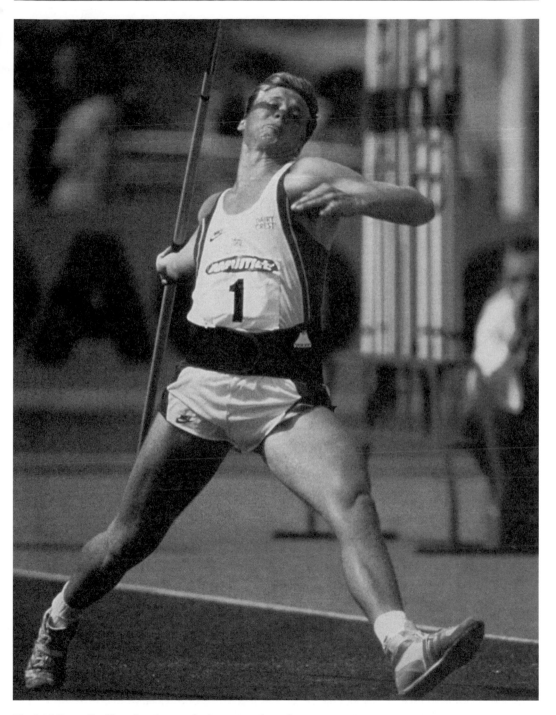

Fig 164 Steve Backley showing explosive strength and power.

Safety

The first priority in strength training is safety. With this in mind, you should take note of the following principles.

As with all other forms of training, you must warm up thoroughly before strength training. The warm-up should follow the guidelines stated and include flexibility work, which can also be done after the strength work-out.

Whatever the exercise, the correct techniques for lifting must be used, including correct breathing.

Start with sensible resistances (loading) and be sure not to lift heavy weights too soon. Too great a weight with a bad body position can result in an *accident*.

Know about and avoid exercises or body positions which can damage vulnerable parts of the body such as the lower back and the knees.

It is suggested that generally with strength training for women, both the extent and the intensity of loading should be increased more gradually than for men. However, this must depend on the individual, state of training and previous experience.

Exercising should cease whenever sharp pain is experienced in the working muscles or in any joint.

Check that the footing is safe and that there is adequate space. The floor should be even, firm and non-slip.

If equipment is to be used, it must be soundly constructed, regularly checked and maintained.

Expert instruction and supervision should be sought in the techniques and usage of the particular equipment.

Loading

Eventually the load (or resistance) which is used will depend on the type of strength to be developed, but the most practical exercise load to develop general strength in the early stages is a weight which can be raised *ten* times in succession. You should continue to work with this load until *twelve* repetitions can be managed, at which point the weight should be increased so as to reduce the number of possible repetitions to *ten* again.

However, if you are using weights for the very first time, start with a lighter load to allow concentration on the correct technique of lifting. As a guide, use a load which you can lift *correctly* for *twelve* repetitions. This load will differ for each exercise, depending on the strength of the particular muscles in use. Only after two or three sessions should a change be made to a load which can be handled adequately for *ten* repetitions. Then continue as previously described.

These can only be general guidelines in the initial stages and subsequently, as already pointed out, any significant improvement in strength is likely to be achieved by using heavier resistances with fewer repetitions, while muscular endurance improves with low resistance and a larger number of repetitions.

Progression

Try to increase the load you are lifting every two to three weeks, for example, if you are doing repetitions of ten, when you complete twelve on the final set, then increase the load a little.

Frequency

On average, strength training can take place two or three times a week. Each session should last from 30 minutes to one hour. This will, of course, depend on physical condition, what particular achievements are being sought and the speed at which the exercise routines are carried out. A standard session might consist of three sets of each exercise.

Order

You should exercise the large muscle groups first, working towards smaller muscles later. A suggested order would be:

LEGS → CHEST → BACK →
SHOULDERS → ARMS → ABDOMINALS

Speed

This is often a neglected consideration in strength training. The optimum speed of a repetition will vary depending on the muscle group being used and the specific requirements of the sport or activity. If the movement is speeded up, this will make the exercise shorter and less effective as a strength builder. Doing faster repetitions is likely to produce a more dynamic kind of strength, power, mainly through adaptation by the nervous system, the neurogenic effects. It will be the slower movements that will tend to strengthen the muscles and connective tissue more effectively.

Rest

The rest between repetitions should be kept to a minimum and will depend on the use of 'rebound' or the 'counter-movement' effect. It will normally be not more than a second. The rest interval between sets should be from one and a half to two minutes depending on the intensity of the session.

After a session of heavy lifting using particular muscle groups, it is advisable to rest for at least 48 hours, although this period may vary according to your physical condition. But, if strength is concentrated on the chest, abdominals and legs on Monday and Thursday, and on the back, shoulders and arms on Tuesday and Friday, that will give at least 72 hours for each muscle group to recover. This is known as a *split routine*.

Specificity

After the basic strength groundwork has been done, choose exercises which are applicable and specific to your sport in terms of the muscle groups to be used, the types of muscular contraction, the movement patterns and the speed of movement.

METHODS OF STRENGTH TRAINING

There is now a great range of methods of strength training. The most obvious means of strength training is to use either free or machine weights to provide the resistance against which muscles work. The use of machines and free weights is obviously efficient as these have been specifically designed for the purpose. The machines offer comfort and assist considerably with the learning of technique. The weights are marked so that the loading is always known and can be altered quickly within any exercise programme. Free weights, once the techniques have been learned and mastered, have proved their effectiveness over a considerable period of time for athletes at all levels. Again, the weight being lifted is known so progress can be monitored. However, there are many other forms of strength training, such as using body resistance – either your own or a partner's – medicine balls, circuits, and elastic bands. These other forms of strength training are often neglected in favour of weights, but in many instances they can provide a more specific form of training in that the movements can simulate more closely those found in competition, so the training can be more sport-specific and flexible in approach compared to the more limited range of movements dictated by a weights machine.

Table 4 Strength training methods.
Individual body resistance exercises
Body resistance exercises using equipment
Partner resistance exercises
Medicine balls
Circuit training
Plyometrics
Pulleys, springs and elastic bands
Free weights
Exercise machines
Isokinetic training
Isometric training

Table 4 sets out the various types of strength-training methods which now exist.

BODY RESISTANCE EXERCISES

The most easily available form of resistance is the body itself. Although there has been considerable increase in weight training facilities, equipment may not be available or convenient to use for an athlete or groups of athletes. A coach may wish to do some strength work during or after a training session on the field or in a gymnasium with a whole group of players. Therefore, body resistance exercises, as they are called, can be useful. For as long as man has practised exercises, all kinds of body resistance exercises have been used extensively. This form of resistance can be exploited more precisely by altering the resistance with a change of body position, by working more extensively on particular muscle groups and providing forms of training such as strength work using a combination of repetitions and changing resistances. This form of training

can also be developed using a partner, either in co-operation or competitively.

The following section shows how one particular exercise, i.e. push-up, can be developed in terms of variety of exercise and changing resistance. The same approach can be used with any exercise with a little thought and imagination.

Body Resistance Exercises

Individual Use of Body Weight

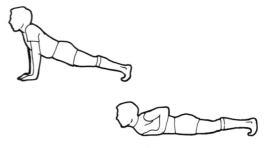

Fig 165.

Push-up (Fig 165) Front support position with arms shoulder width apart; arms bend to lower the chest to the floor and return to front support position. Keep a rigid body throughout.

Push-up on finger tips (Fig 166) Position as above, but resting on finger tips. Follow similar movement.

Push-up slapping chest (Fig 167) Position as above, but push up explosively, touch chest with both hands and then replace hands on floor.

Push-up clapping hands (Fig 168) Position as above, but push up explosively, clap hands and then replace hands on floor.

Push-up feet raised (Fig 169) Position as above, but with feet on a bench. Arms bend

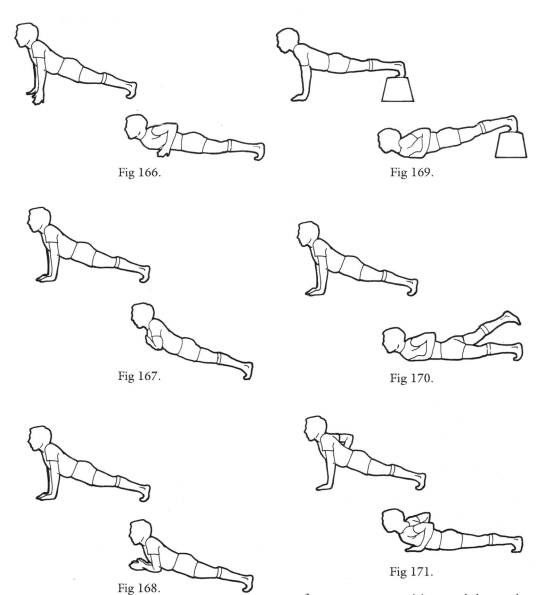

Fig 166.

Fig 169.

Fig 167.

Fig 170.

Fig 171.

Fig 168.

to lower the chest to the floor and return to front support position. Keep a rigid body throughout.

Push-up raising one leg (Fig 170) Position as above. As the arms bend to lower the chest to the floor, raise one leg into the air; return to front support position and lower leg. Repeat with other leg and keep alternating.

One arm push-up (Fig 171) Adopt a balanced position taking support on one arm; arm bends to lower the chest to the floor and return to front support position. Alternate right then left arms.

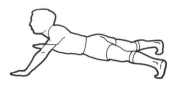

Fig 172.

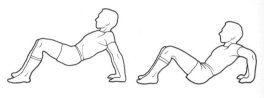

Fig 174.

Extension push-up (Fig 172) Front support position extending arms and feet out wide to the side; arms bend to lower the chest to the floor and return to front support position.

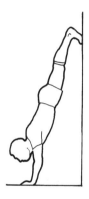

Fig 173.

Push-up from handstand (Fig 173) Handstand position with feet resting on a wall; arms bend to lower forehead to the floor and return to front support position.

Dips (Fig 174) Knees bent, feet flat on the ground, seat just above the floor, arms straight, palms on the floor and fingers pointing forwards; bend the arms as much as possible until your seat touches the floor, then straighten your arms to return to starting position.

Co-operating with a Partner

Combined push-up (Fig 175) Partner A adopts front support position; partner B also adopts front support position with his/her feet on A's shoulders. Both bend arms and lower chests to the floor and return to front support position at the same time.

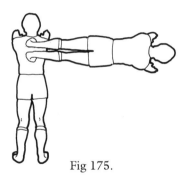

Fig 175.

Push-up feet raised (Fig 176) Partner holds athlete's feet by his calves; athlete presses from full extensions of arms to touch the floor with his chest.

Competing with a Partner

Separate wrists (Fig 177) Partners face one another. Partner A holds arms out in front with elbows bent and palms on top of one another; partner B grips A's wrists and attempts *slowly* to pull them sideways and apart. Partner A tries to keep palms on top of one another.

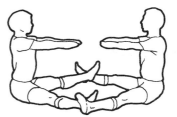

Fig 178.

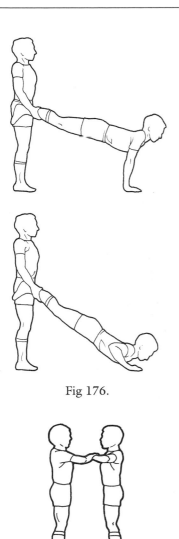

Fig 176.

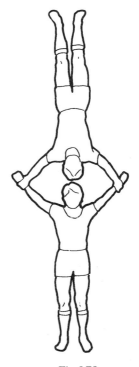

Fig 179.

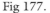

Fig 177.

Separate legs (Fig 178) Partners sit facing each other with feet astride and A's feet just inside B's; A attempts to force legs apart, but B tries to keep legs together.

Clap hands (Fig 179) Partners lie on back with tops of heads together and arms out to the sides. Partner A has palms facing upward and partner B grips A's wrists; A attempts to raise his arms slowly and clap his hands together but B tries to keep A's arms near the floor.

Stand upright (Fig 180) Partners sit back to back with arms interlocked and knees bent with feet placed firmly on the floor. Partner A

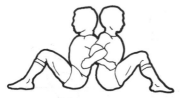

Fig 180.

tries to press with the legs and raise his/her body from the floor; partner B attempts to keep his/her seat on the floor.

Using Beams

Pull-up (overgrasp) (Fig 181) Overgrasp on a beam; pull up to touch beam with chin, then lower to full elbow extension.

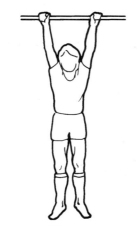

Fig 181.

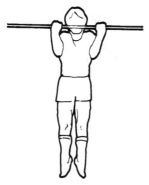

Fig 182.

Pull-up (undergrasp) (Fig 182) Position and exercise as above, but use undergrasp grip.

Pull-up with bent legs (Fig 183) Position as above, but with knees in front of chest.

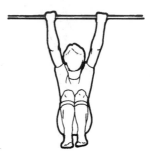

Fig 183.

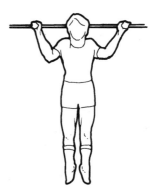

Fig 184.

Heaves to back of neck (Fig 184) Wide overgrasp on a beam or bar with head forward and neck flexed; pull up to back of neck.

Using Ropes

Rope climb (Fig 185) Take hold of rope above head; climb rope using hands and feet.

Rope climb without using feet (Fig 186) Position as above, but climb rope using hands only.

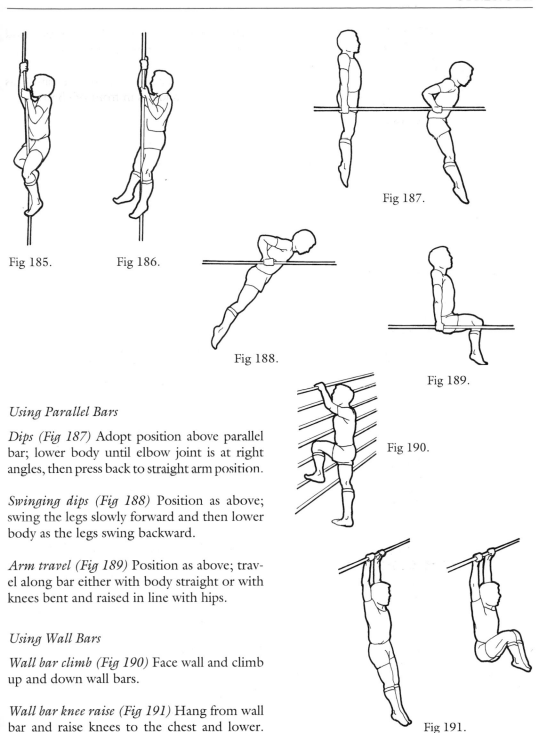

Fig 185.

Fig 186.

Fig 187.

Fig 188.

Fig 189.

Fig 190.

Fig 191.

Using Parallel Bars

Dips (Fig 187) Adopt position above parallel bar; lower body until elbow joint is at right angles, then press back to straight arm position.

Swinging dips (Fig 188) Position as above; swing the legs slowly forward and then lower body as the legs swing backward.

Arm travel (Fig 189) Position as above; travel along bar either with body straight or with knees bent and raised in line with hips.

Using Wall Bars

Wall bar climb (Fig 190) Face wall and climb up and down wall bars.

Wall bar knee raise (Fig 191) Hang from wall bar and raise knees to the chest and lower.

Against a Wall

Static sitting (Fig 192) Sit with back flat against a wall, and knees at 90 degrees. Maintain the position for set time intervals or until fatigue sets in.

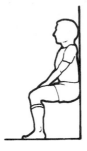

Fig 192.

MEDICINE BALL

Introduction

Medicine ball exercises involve movements of the trunk which are lateral, horizontal or vertical, supported by movement involving the shoulders, arms, hips and legs. The movements should be explosive in nature with an eccentric (pre-stretching or gathering) phase. It is important to get a feel for the rhythm of these exercises. The number of sets and repetitions will, of course, vary for each individual, but as a guide 3–6 sets of 8–15 repetitions on each exercise would be a recommended range, with about one-minute rest intervals between sets. The exercises can be done individually or worked with a partner. As a guide, females can use a 2kg medicine ball and males a 3kg medicine ball, but it will depend on each individual's strength.

Medicine Ball Exercises

Medicine ball throw. In standing position, feet can be either shoulder-width apart *(Fig 193a)*

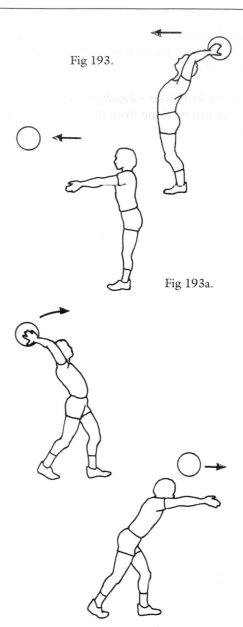

Fig 193.

Fig 193a.

Fig 193b.

or one in front of the other *(Fig 193b)*. Hold the ball firmly on the sides and slightly back, positioning it behind the head with the arms bent. Slowly lean back with the ball behind the head. Powerfully flex the trunk and follow through by throwing the ball out as far as possible. Concentrate on thrusting the arms forward from the shoulders and chest.

Medicine ball throw – kneeling (Fig 194) This exercise can be done from the kneeling position with the knees positioned at about shoulder-width apart. Same action as for Medicine ball throw.

Medicine ball forward swing (Fig 195) Stand with the feet slightly more than shoulder-width apart, the hips flexed and the knees slightly bent, holding the ball between and behind the legs. Swing the ball and toss forwards.

Medicine ball press In standing position with feet either shoulder-width apart (*Fig 196*) or one in front of the other (*Fig 197*) hold the ball at chest height with arms flexed. Push the ball rapidly outwards, extending arms to full length.

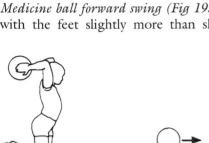

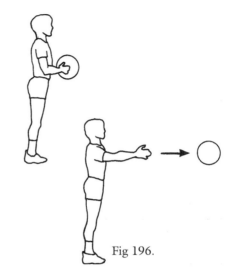

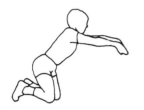

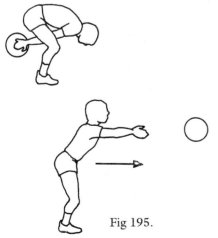

Fig 194.

Fig 196.

Fig 195.

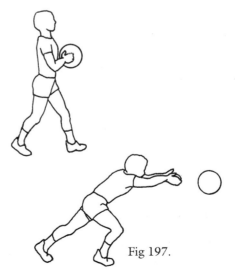

Fig 197.

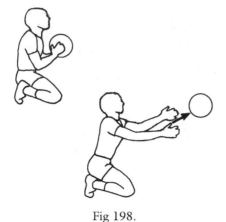

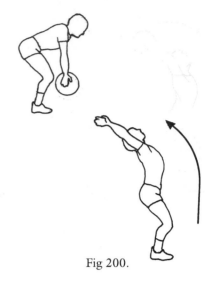

Fig 198.

Fig 200.

Medicine ball press – kneeling (Fig 198) This exercise can be done from the kneeling position with both knees together and the body upright.

Medicine ball toss (Fig 199) Assume a semi-squat position with the ball between the legs, the arms extended, the head held up and the back straight. Begin by pushing the hips forward and moving the shoulders backwards, maintaining full extension of the arms. Toss the ball upwards and forwards, concentrating on fully extending the body.

Medicine ball toss overhead (Fig 200) This exercise can also be done by tossing the ball backwards over the head.

Medicine ball lying throw (Fig 201) Lie flat on the back with the knees bent. Hold the ball behind the head with the arms fully extended. Throw the ball by powerfully flexing from the hips and swinging the arms forwards and upwards.

Medicine ball back swing (Fig 202) Stand with the feet slightly more than shoulder-width apart and the ball above and behind the head. Swing down and toss the ball between the legs.

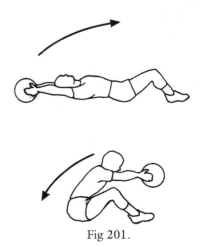

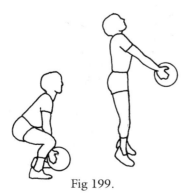

Fig 199.

Fig 201.

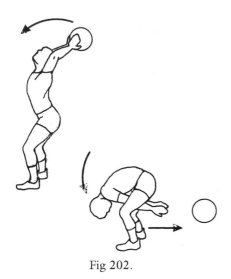

Fig 202.

Medicine ball twist-toss (Fig 203) Hold the ball next to the body at waist level with the feet slightly wider apart than the shoulders. First twist in the direction opposite to the toss, then powerfully twist in the other direction, releasing ball. Use the hips as well as the shoulders and arms.

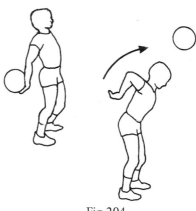

Fig 204.

Medicine ball back-toss (Fig 204) Stand with the feet shoulder-width apart, holding the ball behind the back with the palms facing backwards and the hands underneath the ball. Flip the ball by powerfully extending the arms back and at the same time flexing at the hip.

Medicine ball leg toss (Fig 205) Stand with the ball held firmly between the feet, holding on to a beam above the head. Swing the legs as straight as possible and use the hips to generate most of the force.

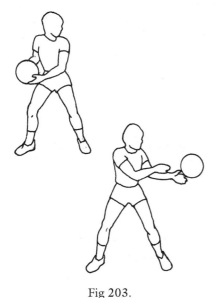

Fig 203.

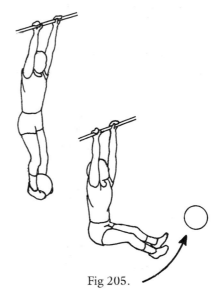

Fig 205.

87

WEIGHT TRAINING

A similar approach to using body weight as resistance is followed in the area of weight training; it is still a matter of finding appropriate resistances against which the muscles of the body can work. If you need to work in the garage at home or in some area close to a training ground, you can use a little inventiveness and imagination in producing suitable equipment. Appropriately weighted and sized iron bars or logs of wood can be used, providing you are conscious of the safety requirements previously outlined. Without question, exercise machines and good quality free weights are the best answer, but we should never forget the basic notion of strength work, where a muscle or group of muscles contracts *against increasing resistance.*

Many gyms and fitness centres consist mainly of exercise machines because of their attractive design and comfort and because they can be used with less supervision. However, with exercise machines, and particularly free weights, qualified instruction is required for the beginner and then continuous monitoring of training should take place.

Most machines use weight for resistance in the form of an adjustable stack or carriage which can be loaded with plates. Hydraulic cylinders or air pressure are other forms of resistance on machines. Most machines can be accommodated to a variety of body types so an element of comfort is provided. With free weights in addition to barbells and dumb-bells, there is additional equipment such as benches and squat racks. Generally, weight training exercises using free weights will be more effective and efficient, if the technique is sound, in developing strength.

The following section outlines some core weight training exercises (*see also* Table 5)

Table 5 Core exercises.	
Legs	1. **Power Clean**
	2. **Back Squat**
	3. **Front Squat**
	4. **Hamstring Curl**
	5. **High Pull**
Chest	6. **Bench Press**
	7. **Dumb-Bell Flyes**
Back	8. **Lat Pull Down**
Shoulder	9. **Military Press**
	10. **Press behind Neck**
Arms	11. **Bicep Curl**
	12. **Tricep Extension**
	13. **Lateral Dumb-Bell Raise**
Abdominals	14. *see* page 95

incorporating the main starting and lifting positions which are very important. The recommended procedures and techniques are included but as stated earlier you will need to seek the right guidance and supervision for the full range of weight-training exercises.

Clean *(Figs 206–208)*

Also known as the power clean, this is a good all-round exercise for all athletes developing leg, back, arm and shoulder strength.

1. Adopt the basic standing start position for most weight training exercises: feet slightly wider than hip-width apart, heels flat on the floor and toes turned slightly outward. Insteps under bar with shins almost touching bar; body standing erect with arms by the sides.

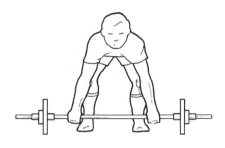

Fig 206.

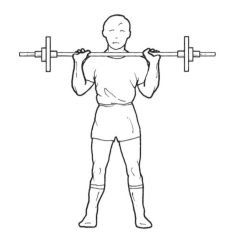

Fig 207.

2. From standing position, bend from the hips and knees to take up a crouch position and grip the bar using an overgrasp grip just wider than shoulder-width apart. Arms should remain straight and relaxed. Look up with back flat and seat as high as the position comfortably permits.

3. Raise the bar by extending the legs and keeping arms fully straight. Keep the bar close to the legs and press the thighs forward as the bar passes the knees. Keep the bar moving continuously close to body, and when bar reaches chest height, drop the hips, while bending at the knees, so lowering shoulder to bar level.

4. Hands and forearms rotate under the bar to place it across the front of the chest with palms upwards in the receiving position. Force the elbows forward to rest the bar on the chest so as to avoid supporting weight of bar with the arms.

5. To return bar to the floor, lower to the thighs, and then to the floor.

6. Breathe *in* during the lift and *out* as the bar is lowered.

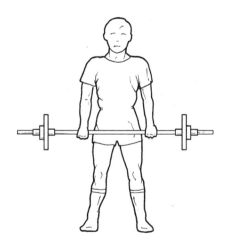

Fig 208.

Military Press *(Figs 209 and 210)*

An exercise for developing arm and shoulder strength.

1. Clean the bar to the chest rest position *(Fig 209)*; this is another important starting position, and is the end position of the clean previously described. As stated, the bar rests on the upper chest with an overgrasp grip slightly more than shoulder-width apart and the hands under the bar. Elbows are flexed

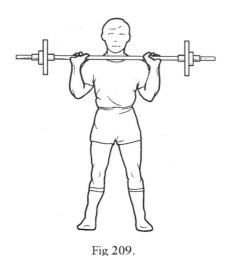

Fig 209.

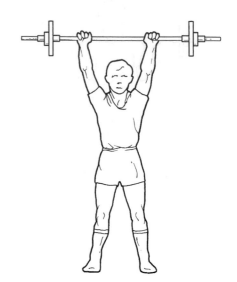

Fig 210.

and pointing forward; legs and back are straight with feet placed comfortably slightly wider than a hip-width apart.

2. From this starting position, press the bar to full arm extension directly above the head. Keep legs and back straight throughout (*Fig 210*).

3. Breathe *in* on pressing the bar and *out* on lowering.

Bicep Curl *(Figs 211 and 212)*

An exercise for strengthening the flexors of the arms.

1. The next basic starting position is used for this exercise, the thigh support position. Adopt a standing position with shoulders pulled back; arms fully extended gripping bar (for curl, an undergrasp) resting against the thighs.

2. From this position, raise the bar by slowly flexing the arms until the bar reaches the chest, keeping the elbows still and against the side of the trunk. Keep head up throughout

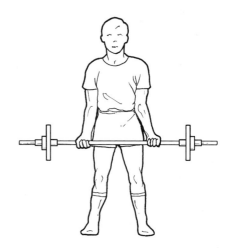

Fig 211.

exercise. Then lower bar slowly back to starting position.

3. Breathe *in* when lifting bar and *out* when lowering.

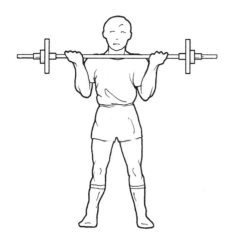

Fig 212.

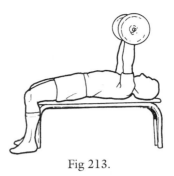

Fig 213.

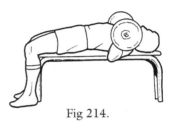

Fig 214.

Bench Press *(Figs 213 and 214)*

A major exercise for strengthening the arms and shoulders. It is also of general use for upper body development.

1. Bench press is an exercise which requires the use of support racks or two helpers (spotters) with clear communication between the athlete and the spotters at the beginning and the end of the exercise.
2. Assume a lying position (on your back) on the bench. Feet resting firmly on the ground, knees bent at right angles with feet turned slightly outward; this is the supine starting position.
3. Before taking the bar from the racks or spotters, the hands, using overgrasp, should be positioned on the bar so it is well balanced and the arms outstretched above the upper chest.
4. With the palms under and supporting the bar, take the weight and lower under control to the chest, then press upward to fully straighten the arms.

5. Breathe *in* when lowering the bar and *out* as the arms straighten.

Back Squat *(Figs 215–218)*

This exercise is a good strengthener of the legs, back and chest.

1. Adopt the shoulder rest starting position with feet slightly wider than hip-width apart; bar is behind neck, resting across shoulders and back of neck. Head up and shoulders braced back; an overgrasp grip with hands more than shoulder width apart and elbows flexed.
2. Maintain a flat, upright back. Lower hips and bar by bending the legs while pushing the knees outwards. Keep the back as flat as possible and keep the head pressed back. Control the downward movement until the thighs are

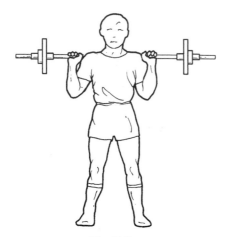

Fig 215.

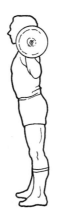

Fig 216.

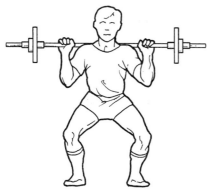

Fig 217.

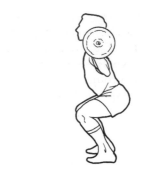

Fig 218.

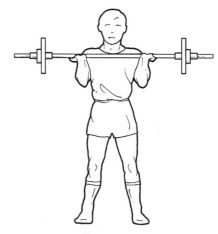

Fig 219.

parallel to the floor (it is inadvisable to lower further).

3. Powerfully lift the weight back to the starting position, straighten the legs and press the hips forward under the bar in order to maintain a strong lifting position.

4. Breathe *in* on lowering and *out* on lifting.

Front Squat *(Fig 219)*

The starting position is as for the back squat but the bar is now resting across the front of the shoulders and the top of the chest, with the elbows held high and hands slightly wider than shoulder-width apart.

The action is the same as for the back squat. This exercise develops leg, hip and back strength and it places greater demands on the quadriceps than the back squat. It exercises the main muscle groups; quadriceps, gluteus maximus, erector spinae, biceps brachii.

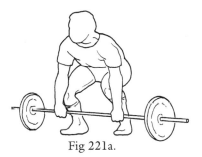

Fig 221a.

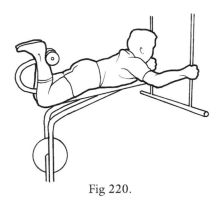

Fig 220.

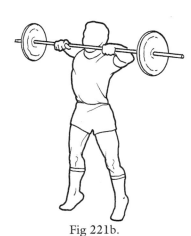

Fig 221b.

Hamstring Curl *(Fig 220)*

1. Lie face down on the bench with the backs of the ankles under the higher padded roll. Grip the bars with both hands. The head should be raised comfortably and the spine as flat as possible.
2. Lift the heels and pull the bar towards the buttocks as far as possible.
3. Slowly lower the weight back down to the starting position, where the hamstrings are comfortably stretched.
4. Breathe *in* as the knees flex and *out* as they extend to lower the weight down.

High Pull *(Fig 221)*

1. Starting position as for the clean *(Fig 221a)*.
2. Raise the bar by extending the legs powerfully, then rise on the toes as the bar is pulled to the chin in one smooth movement *(Fig 221b)*.

Dumb-Bell Flyes *(Figs 222 and 223)*

1. The starting position is as for the bench press, holding the dumb-bells vertically above the chest with arms fully extended and the palms of the hands facing each other.
2. Bending the elbows, slowly lower the weights down to the sides.
3. Pull the dumb-bells back to the starting position.
4. Breathe *in* as the weights are lowered and breathe *out* as the weights are brought upwards.

This exercise strengthens the shoulder horizontal flexors. Main muscle groups: pectorals and deltoids.

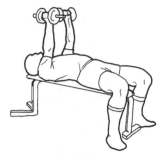

Fig 222.

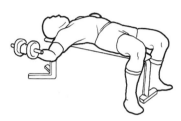

Fig 223.

and bring the bar just below the chin.

3. Allow the weight to return by slowly letting the bar rise back to the start position.

4. Breathe *in* as you pull down and breathe *out* as the weight is controlled back.

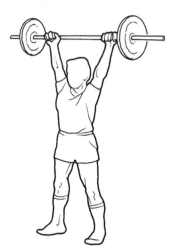

Fig 225.

Lat Pull Down *(Fig 224)*

1. Sit securely on the seat, allowing the spine to stretch fully with the bar above the head. Use the wide overgrasp on the bar.

2. Slowly pull the bar down in front of the face. Draw elbows downwards to the sides

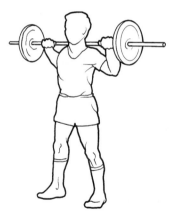

Fig 226.

Press behind Neck *(Figs 225 and 226)*

1. The starting position is as for the military press but hold the bar across the back of the neck and shoulders.

2. Press upwards to a full arm extension directly above the head. As with the military

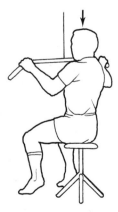

Fig 224.

press, maintain good balance and control, keeping the legs and back straight.
3. Lower the bar slowly and carefully back to rest on the back of the neck and shoulders.
4. Breathe *in* on pressing the bar and breathe *out* on lowering the bar.

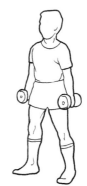

Fig 228.

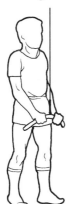

Fig 227.

Tricep Extension *(Fig 227)*

1. Take hold of the bar using an overgrasp grip. The stance should be comfortable with the back straight.
2. Push the bar down to arm's length with the elbows tucked close into the sides of the body.
3. Control the bar back to the starting position.
4. Breathe *in* as the bar is pushed down and breathe *out* as it is brought back to the starting position.

Lateral Dumb-Bell Raise
(Figs 228 and 229)

1. Stand with the feet slightly more than hip-width apart. Hold a dumb-bell in each hand with the palms facing inwards.
2. Keeping the arms straight, raise the dumb-bells sideways to a position where the weights are slightly higher than shoulder level. Do not swing the weight, use the shoulders.

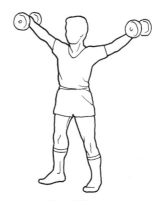

Fig 229.

Abdominals

It is vital that the abdominals are not neglected in any training programme. They have a dual role in either causing movement – for example, flexing the trunk – or for stability, by holding the spine firm. So in sport they are involved in actions which move the trunk, often dynamically, and at the same time have a stabilizing function in controlling trunk alignment and movement. The abdominals also form the 'pillar' off which the upper body operates. So overall they play a key role in providing core stability and causing a range of movement. There is a range of abdominal muscles operating

95

vertically, diagonally and horizontally, so it is important to use a range of exercises to work all the main abdominal muscles.

The exercises should be performed lying on the back with knees bent (at 90 degrees) and feet flat on the floor (unless otherwise indicated) unanchored. The hands should be placed on the shoulders with arms folded across the chest and elbows pointing forwards.

Start with sets of ten to twenty and build up to sets of thirty on each exercise.

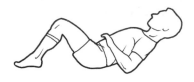

Fig 232.

Bent Legs Hands Between Legs (Fig 233)

Curl up and place hands between legs.

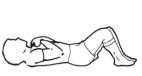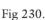

Fig 230.

Abdominal Curl (Fig 230)

Lie on back with knees bent and hands across chest; raise trunk and touch both knees with elbows.

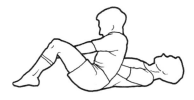

Fig 233.

Bent Legs Elbows to Thighs (Fig 231)

Curl up to place right elbow on left knee, and on next repetition left elbow on right knee.

Bent Legs Opposite Ankle on Knee (Fig 234)

Place ankle on top of opposite knee. Curl up and twist towards knee; change to other ankle and knee and repeat movement.

Bent Legs Curl Up and Twist Low (Fig 232)

Curl up a short distance and twist to touch elbow on the floor.

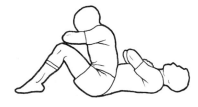

Fig 231.

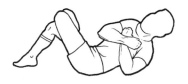

Fig 234.

Bent Legs on Toes (Fig 235)

Press toes into ground and raise heels. Curl up to place elbows on thighs.

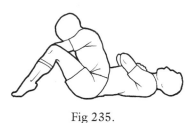

Fig 235.

Knee Raise (Fig 236)

Lie on back with legs straight and arms beside body. Bring knees to chest and then back to starting position.

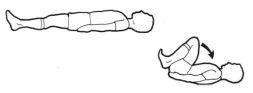

Fig 236.

Bent Legs with Knees at Right Angles (Fig 237)

Raise up feet so that knees are at right angles with lower legs out straight. Curl up to place elbows on thighs

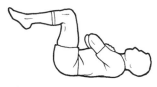

Fig 237.

Knee and Chest Raise (Fig 238)

Position as above. Raise trunk and bring knees to chest at the same time.

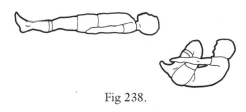

Fig 238.

Reverse Crunches (Fig 239)

Raise up feet so that lower legs are off the ground. Keeping back and head on floor, bring knees towards chest.

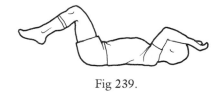

Fig 239.

Twist Crunches (Fig 240)

Sit in crunch position with feet raised so that lower legs are off the ground and straight. Curl up and twist to touch opposite knee with elbow whilst keeping shoulders off the floor.

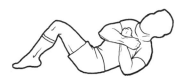

Fig 240.

Double Crunches (Fig 241)

Put one foot on the opposite knee and curl this knee towards the chest whilst moving your chest towards the knee.

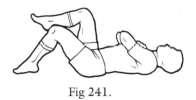

Fig 241.

STRENGTH TRAINING PROGRAMME

In order to obtain a structure and progression to your strength training it is useful to plan the sessions and complete a weight training card which enables you to record and monitor progress. The following sessions are examples of using machine or free weights, but this form of strength training can be supplemented by using body resistance, medicine balls, plyometrics, etc.

Session 1

In the early stages of strength training select a variety of exercises which work on the main muscle groups and adopt the recommended order: legs – chest – back – shoulders – arms – abdominals.

Select ten exercises and establish your ten repetition maximum (10RM) on each exercise. This is the maximum load which you can lift repeatedly on, say, bench press ten times without rest. When the first set of ten exercises (ten repetitions on each) has been achieved, after a short rest (1½–2 minutes), repeat with another set and eventually with a third set. An alternative way would be to increase the number of sets on each exercise before moving to the next. For example, two sets of ten repetitions on front squat, then two sets of ten repetitions on leg press. This can be increased to three sets of ten repetitions on each exercise.

Session 2

Select eight to ten exercises and establish your ten repetitions maximum. On each exercise perform three sets of ten repetitions (a short rest of 1½–2 minutes between each set): the first set at 50 per cent of 10RM (say 12.5kg); the second set with 75 per cent of 10RM (say 19kg); and the third set with the full 10RM (say 25kg). As soon as you can lift twelve repetitions or more for the final set it no longer represents the 10RM and a new heavier load should be adopted.

Session 3

Select eight exercises and establish your 1RM on each exercise. This is the maximum load which you can lift once only on each exercise. Perform six to eight repetitions 75–85 per cent of 1RM on each exercise. Three to four sets with a two minutes' recovery between sets.

Session 4

Select six to ten exercises and establish your 2RM, the maximum load you can lift twice. This session involves increasing the loads successively in each set while the number per set is reduced. For example, on power clean one set could be: seven reps at 15kg; six reps at 20kg; five reps at 25kg; four reps at 30kg; three reps at 35kg; two reps at 40kg. The increase in load could be 2.5kg or 5kg as shown, depending on strength level and previous training.

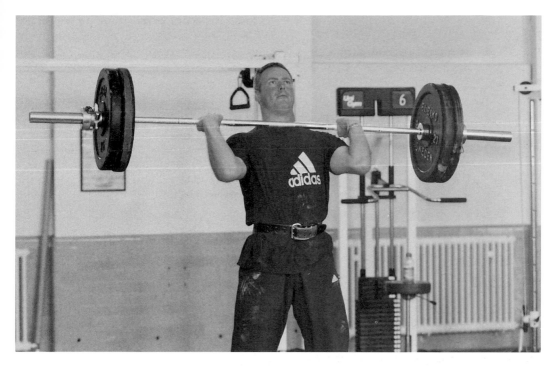

Fig 242 An athlete using free weights to develop strength and power.

Session 5

Select six to ten exercises and establish your 1RM on each exercise. For set 1 – five reps at 75 per cent of 1RM; set 2 – four reps at 80 per cent of 1RM; set 3 – three reps at 80–85 per cent of 1RM; set 4 – two reps at 85–90 per cent of 1RM; set 5 – one rep at 95–100 per cent of 1RM; 2 minutes' rest between sets.

Session 6

Select six to ten exercises and establish your 1RM on each exercise: set 1 – five reps at 75 per cent of 1RM; set 2 – three reps at 80–85 per cent of 1RM; set 3 – one rep at 95–100 per cent of 1RM; set 4 – three reps at 80–85 per cent of 1RM; set 5 – five reps at 75 per cent of 1RM; two minutes' recovery between sets.

Session 7

Select six to ten exercises and establish your 1RM on each exercise. Try to perform two to three sets at each weight resistance, either rotating round the exercises or on one at a time. Set 1 – three reps at fifty per cent of 1RM; set 2 – three reps at 60 per cent of 1RM; set 3 – three reps at 70 per cent of 1RM; set 4 – three reps at 80 per cent of 1RM; set 5 – three reps at 90 per cent of 1RM; one minute's recovery between sets.

Session 8

Select four to eight exercises and establish your 1RM on each exercise. Try to perform two sets at each weight resistance. Set 1 – six reps at 50 per cent of 1RM; set 2 – five reps at 60 per cent of 1RM.; set 3 – three reps at

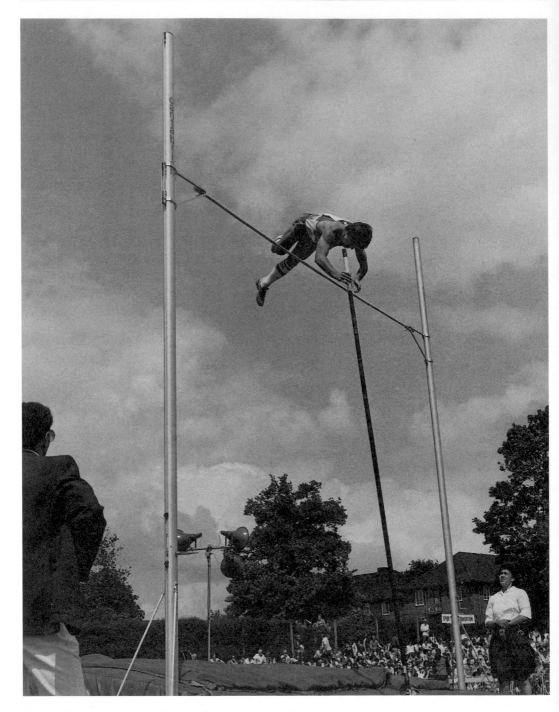

Fig 243 Pole vault: a test of strength, power and technique.

70 per cent of 1 RM; set 4 – two reps at 80 per cent of 1 RM; set 5 – one rep at 90 per cent of 1 RM; set 6 – two reps at 80 per cent of 1 RM; set 7 – three reps at 70 per cent of 1 RM; one minute's recovery between sets.

Session 9

Select six to eight exercises and establish your 6RM on each exercise (the maximum weight which you can lift six times). Follow this procedure for each exercise in turn: perform six repetitions or as many as you can until fatigue; rest for two minutes; perform as many repetitions as you can (this could be less than previous set); rest for two minutes; perform as many repetitions as you can (this could be less than the previous two sets because of fatigue); two minutes' rest; move to next exercise and repeat.

Session 10

Select six to eight exercises and establish your 6RM on each exercise. Follow this procedure for each exercise in turn: perform two repetitions; one minute's rest; perform four repetitions; one minute's rest; perform six repetitions or as many repetitions until fatigue; two minutes' rest; two repetitions; two minutes' rest; move to next exercise and repeat.

All forms of training should be planned over a lengthy period of time. Any physiological adaptations that take place as a result of training will occur over an extended period. In addition, most of the adaptations which result from hard training are reversible, so any period of inactivity will cause a decline in strength; fitness is hard to gain and easy to lose. Sound preparation for a particular sport involves planning a cyclical year-round programme. There will be considerable variation between sports, but generally each sport

will have a competitive season of a certain length. Consequently, the training should be divided into phases, with an out-of-season phase, pre-season phase (preparation), and a competition phase.

You will need to develop a varied and progressive strength programme based on these divisions. In strength training, the aim would be to achieve a balanced ratio of *general strength*, *specialized strength* and *competition based strength*. The following represents a guideline but there will be considerable variation between individual athletes and the particular demands of their sport.

Cyclical Programme

During the out-of-season phase the aim would be to develop general strength. The schedules would be general in nature, employing major exercises for all muscle groups. The major objective would be to achieve a balanced development and the establishment of a sound basis for the strength work to follow. Repetitions will be high and there will be a gradual increase in weight.

As you move into the pre-season phase, the training decreases in the general area as specialized strength exercises are increased. These exercises take individual components of the sport technique and develop those components in accordance with the type of strength required. Sets of varying repetitions and weights, for example a pyramid method, are most appropriate at this stage.

During the competition phase the aim should be to maintain levels of specialized strength developed in the previous phase while incorporating competition-based exercises which are closely related to the techniques of your sport.

A possible dosage of two or three strength sessions per week could be pursued in the

101

out-of-season and pre-season phases. Maintenance is then a key factor, although with such long playing seasons (up to nine months) strength gains are possible just as endurance can be improved over the competitive season. However, it is important to structure strength sessions around match days and team training in order for the body to recover and adapt effectively.

Strength development has been consistently shown to have a significant influence in the performance of several sports, although the programme will not contain all the answers to training. It must be carefully planned to complement and fit similar programmes for flexibility, speed, endurance, and so on.

POWER

The importance of power in many sports cannot be stressed enough and it is a vital quality in successful performance. Power is defined physically as force multiplied by velocity, but a simpler and more appropriate definition for sport would be strength with speed. As a consequence there will always be a close relationship between strength and power work. Strength is a primary prerequisite for power, so a programme aimed at developing power must first concentrate on improving strength. Once strength has been developed speed of movement, rather than the resistance, is the key factor.

It is possible to do power work using weights in the form of weights machines, free weights and dumb-bells. The same weight training programme can be used and this has the advantage that the athlete is familiar with the technique. This is a considerable advantage because speed of movement is required. This speed has to be under control and exercises chosen that allow explosive movement to be performed efficiently. The movement

needs to be at a certain speed in order to recruit the fast-twitch fibres which are the ones responsible for the fast explosive movements. As in all strength training the amount of resistance is crucial and in this case it has to allow a fast, controlled movement whilst providing a resistance to the contracting muscle. In order to achieve this a resistance of between 60 and 80 per cent of 1RM would be suitable to perform power weights.

Before performing any power-weight sessions, make sure you are fully warmed up and have stretched properly. Select about three to six exercises per session and do ten repetitions on each exercise and one to three sets of each. The emphasis is on quality and speed of movement.

Suggested exercises for power weights:

Power Clean
Bench Press
Shoulder Press
Lat Pull Down
Pec Deck
Cable Pulls
Triceps Extension.

PLYOMETRICS

Many athletes who have undertaken extensive weight training programmes have found that the increase of strength developed did not always transfer to the performance in improving the quality needed. A possible answer to this would be the use of plyometric training.

Plyometrics are training drills which are designed to develop that quality in the athlete which bridges the gap between sheer strength and the power required to produce explosive reactive movements shown very clearly in activities like jumping, throwing and sprinting.

The basic thinking behind this particular approach to training is that maximum tension develops when active muscle is stretched quickly. The faster a muscle is forced to lengthen, the greater the tension it exerts. The rate of stretch is more important than the magnitude of stretch. The greater a muscle is pre-stretched from its natural length in the body before contraction occurs, the greater load the muscle will be able to lift. In other words, a concentric contraction of a muscle (shortening) is much stronger if it immediately follows an eccentric contraction (lengthening or pre-stretching) of the same muscle. The word 'immediately' is important, for to achieve optimum results from the pre-stretching of an eccentric contraction, the effects of which are of very short duration, the subsequent concentric contraction must take place within fractions of a second. What are the explanations for the increased force of which a muscle can exert concentrically (while shortening) immediately after it contracts eccentrically (lengthens)? As the muscle is being pre-stretched and lengthened during the eccentric phase, the 'slack' is taken up during this gathering or amortization phase. In addition, the stretch or myotatic reflex can cause higher contraction values when preceded by stretching in the muscle, as there is stimulation of the stretch receptors or muscle spindles during stretching which cause proprioceptive nerve impulses to travel to the spinal cord and return to the same muscle causing a powerful contraction to prevent *overstretching* of the muscle. Finally, at the end of the eccentric phase (the pre-stretching), elastic energy is stored in the 'elastic' elements of the muscle. Stretch a rubber band to one quarter of its possible stretch length, then stretch it to three-quarters of its possible length – it will snap back more forcefully when stretched further.

Plyometric exercises are used to train the eccentric aspect of muscle action. Many athletes have tremendous strength but they are often unable to produce the *power* necessary in explosive activities. They fail to bridge the gap between sheer strength and power. Plyometric work seeks to bridge this gap.

When designing plyometric exercises, certain factors should be considered:

1. Maximum tension develops when active muscle is stretched quickly.
2. The faster a muscle is forced to lengthen, the greater the tension it exerts.
3. The rate of stretch is more important than the magnitude of stretch.
4. Utilize the overload principle, which specifies that increased strength results only from work performed at an intensity greater than that to which it is accustomed.

Considerable care should be taken in developing the use of these exercises in the early stages as they can present noticeable stress to joints like the knee.

Plyometric Drills

Warm-up properly and ensure that you are thoroughly warm and stretched prior to any plyometric drills.

LOWER BODY

Concentrate on quality. Drills must be done with maximum effort. Ensure you have recovered fully from any prior drills.

Squat Jump (Fig 244)

With feet placed about shoulder-width apart and hands down by the sides, begin the movement by quickly lowering to a half-squat position, then check this downward movement by exploding upwards as high as possible and throwing the arms upwards to assist the take-off. Upon landing repeat the

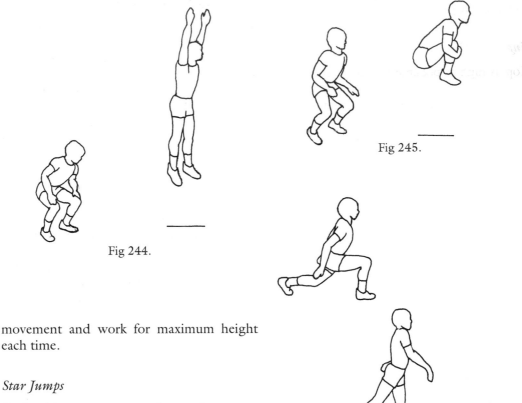

Fig 244.

Fig 245.

Fig 246.

movement and work for maximum height each time.

Star Jumps

Begin this movement as the previous exercise, lower to half-squat position and then check the movement by exploding upwards as high as possible and extending the limbs outward in all four directions away from the body. Immediately on landing repeat the movement and work for maximal height each time.

Knee Tuck (Fig 245)

With the feet comfortably apart, lower the body by bending the knees then, keeping the arms by the sides, drive upwards so that the knees reach near to the chest. Upon landing repeat the movement, trying to drive the knees towards the chest on each repetition.

Split Jump (Fig 246)

Stand with one foot forward and the other to the rear, with the front knee bent at 90 degrees and a slight bend in the rear leg. Jump up as high as possible and in mid-air change the legs over quickly from front to back and back to front before landing. The arms also change to maintain balance. Upon landing repeat the movement, changing over the position of the legs.

Single Leg Hops

Hop as high as possible for about 10m. Use the non-standing leg to try and maximize the length of each hop and work for maximum height.

Running Bounding

Exaggerate the normal running action so that the arms are driven back and through, the knees are lifted high and the back leg drives forcefully from the floor. Work for maximum height from each stride and upon landing spring immediately into the next stride and repeat for 15m.

Double Leg Bound (Fig 247)

Stand with the feet comfortably apart and knees bent in the half-squat position, arms at the side and shoulders forward over the knees. Jump forward and upwards, driving from the hips and knees whilst swinging the arms forward. Try to get as much height as possible and straighten the body in the air. Upon landing bend the knees and repeat the movement.

Alternate Leg Bound (Fig 248)

Stand with one foot slightly in front of the other and the arms at the sides. Push off with the back leg, driving the knee up in front of the chest and trying to get as high as possible. Repeat the movement by driving with

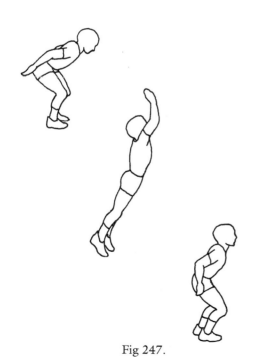

Fig 247.

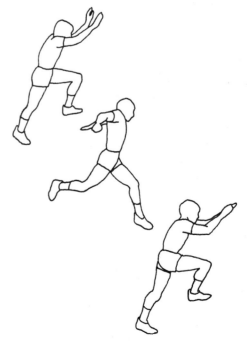

Fig 248.

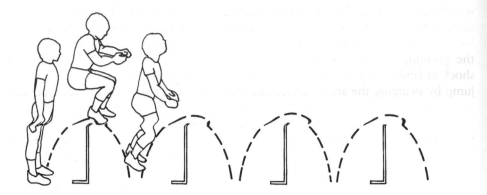

Fig 249.

the other foot on landing. The arms change in co-ordination with the leg movements to maintain balance and continuity of movement.

Double Leg Hurdle Jump (Fig 249)

This exercise requires a set of hurdles of appropriate height about a metre apart. Face the first hurdle with the feet comfortably apart. Begin by lowering the body, then jump explosively with both feet together and keeping the knees high over the first hurdle. On landing continue the movements over the remaining hurdles, concentrating on driving the knees upwards and swinging the arms forwards.

Depth Jump (Fig 250)

This exercise requires two to four boxes placed about a metre apart. Stand on the first box

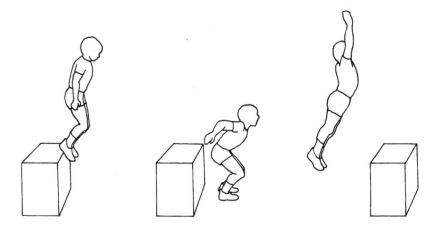

Fig 250.

with the knees slightly bent and the arms at the sides. Drop from the position on the box to land with both feet together. On contact with the ground, bend the knees to absorb the shock of landing and immediately initiate the jump by swinging the arms upward and driving up as powerfully as possible to land on the surface of the next box. Continue this movement over any further boxes.

Cone Jumps

Use 30cm-high cones placed half a metre apart. Two cones mark a line 5m away *(Fig 251)*.

1. Double-footed hops over cones and upon final landing sprint 5m to line.

2. One-footed hops over cones and sprint 5m on landing; alternate left and right.

3. Side hops over cones and turn on final hop to face forward and sprint 5m. Lead with left and right leg alternately.

4. Side hops over cones, then side hops back to first cone, then side hops forward again, to sprint 5m.

5. Side hops over first two cones then turn 180 degrees over third cone, sideways hop back with another 180 degree turn over last cone, then sideways hop over cones, turn and sprint 5m.

Change position of cones as shown for following exercise *(Fig 252)*.

6. Double-footed hops diagonally over cones then sprint 5m.

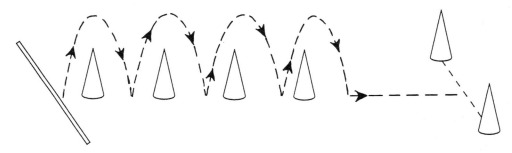

Fig 251.

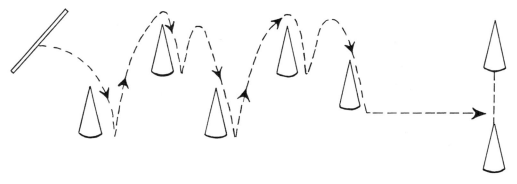

Fig 252.

Stair Jumps

Using suitable steps or stairs (for example, in a stadium or on a spectator's stand): double or single leg bounds (alternating left and right), jumping forwards and upwards, driving from the hips and the knees. This can also be done sideways, alternating left and right feet in single leg bounds.

UPPER BODY

Plyometric Push-up

Front support position with chest on the ground. Push up off the ground so that both the hands and the legs completely leave the ground. On landing back on the ground push up again quickly with feet and hands.

Dumb-Bell Horizontal Swing (Fig 253)

Stand with the feet shoulder-width apart and the arms extended out in front of the chest, holding a dumb-bell of suitable weight in both hands. Pull the dumb-bell to one side and allow the trunk to twist. At the end of the swing quickly check the movement and pull the dumb-bell in the other direction. Continue these movements from side to side.

Dumb-Bell Alternate Arm Swing (Fig 254)

Stand with the feet comfortably apart and the knees slightly bent, holding a dumb-bell of suitable weight in each hand. Swing one arm forwards and upwards to above the shoulder while taking the other arm backwards. Check the movement at the end of each swing and reverse the direction.

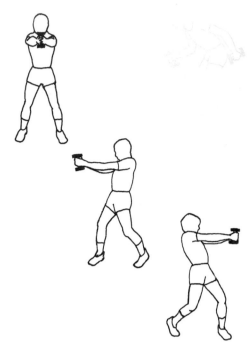

Fig 253.

Dumb-Bell Vertical Swing (Fig 255)

Stand with the feet shoulder-width apart, knees bent, and hold a dumb-bell of suitable weight (or other suitable object) in both hands between the legs. Keep the back straight and the head up. Swing the dumb-bell upwards, keeping the arms straight and letting the body extend. At the top of the swing quickly change direction and pull the dumb-bell down. Keep repeating these movements continuously.

These are a few examples of plyometric exercises. When this type of training is used, basic work employing the kind of exercises described above should be carried out but should also include some specific plyometric drills which

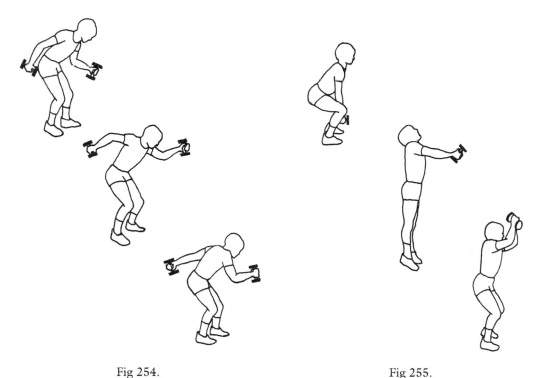

Fig 254.   Fig 255.

are designed to meet the demands of particular sports. If working with a group or team the exercises can be set in the form of a circuit in a gymnasium.

Plyometric Circuit *(Fig 256)*

1. Alternate hopping over a distance of 5 metres; driving back with other foot and driving for distance; use of arms; trotting back to start.
2. Deep squat jumps holding on to a beam.
3. Astride jumps over a gymnasium bench; bend into crouch and drive.
4. Squat thrusts; stretch and extend in long position; movement to be explosive.

5. Depth jumps; jump from a vaulting box to land on mat followed immediately by explosive jump on to a vaulting box; from this position repeat depth jump to next vaulting box.
6. High jumping bringing knees to chest.

Suggested organization; one minute on each exercise; one minute rest interval.

Note The manner in which each exercise is done is important. The muscles being worked should be pre-stretched followed immediately by a rapid contraction, so timing of movement is important. also, in the rest intervals the muscles should be stretched using a range of flexibility exercises.

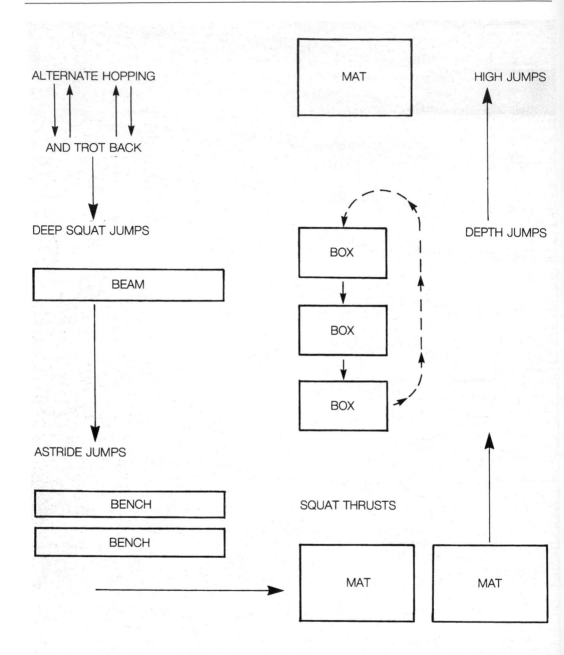

Fig 256 Layout of plyometric circuit.

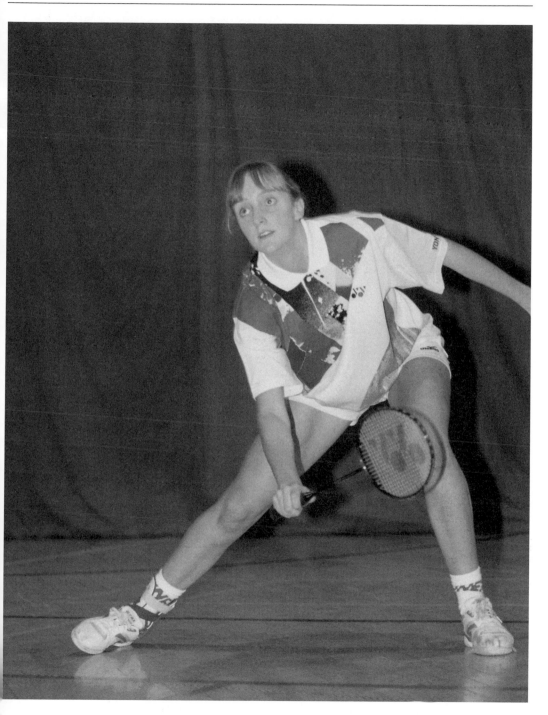

Fig. 257 Badminton requires speed and power.

CHAPTER 6
Speed

DEVELOPMENT OF SPEED

Speed is a major component in many sports, although the actual nature and function will vary. Maximum running speed is essential for sprinters in athletics and for wingers in a number of field games, although optimal speed may be more important in control situations. In addition, speed of limb may be a critical factor in such activities as fast bowling in cricket and serving in tennis, rather than whole body speed. As with other components of fitness, the relative contribution and nature of speed varies according to the particular requirements of the sport, and the speed characteristic is closely associated with other components, particularly strength and flexibility.

It is often considered that speed is an innate quality, that some people are born to be fast. There is probably some truth in this, as we all know of young athletes who are good sprinters without training. We also inherit from our parents and ancestors a certain combination of muscle fibre types which may give some people a natural advantage in some activities. As already discussed to some extent earlier, muscle is thought to be composed of different fibre types:

Type I fibres are the slow, 'red' fibres which help us to perform low-intensity exercise for long periods by having a high aerobic capacity for energy supply, and are fatigue resistant but have a low power output and limited potential for rapid force development.

Type IIa fibres are the intermediate fibres which can contribute to both high- and low-intensity work. They have a moderate power output, fatiguability and aerobic endurance. **Type IIb fibres** are the fast 'white' fibres which can develop force rapidly, have a high power output and high fatiguability. Athletes with a higher proportion of Type II fibres could have an advantage in speed and power. Although speed is less susceptible to improvement than endurance and strength, with the appropriate training programme speed can be improved substantially.

Reaction Time/Movement Time

When considering speed work it is logical firstly to focus on the aspects of initial reaction and movement. In a number of sports, particularly games and sprinting, the ability of an athlete to react to the presentation of a stimulus, such as the release of the cricket ball, the movement of an attacker or the sound of the starter's pistol, must be a major influence in the performance. These factors relate to *reaction time* which is the time lapse between the presentation of the stimulus or cue and the first muscular contraction in response. There are a number of considerations concerned with the improvement of reaction time, both psychological and physiological, but reaction time can be improved with practice provided the practice conditions simulate the actual game or sport requirements. A decrease in total response time, which includes reaction time and movement time, over short distances must be of major consideration to all games players.

Initial body position and step pattern will inevitable affect an athlete's ability to respond quickly. When fast movements are required from a standing position, the best stance is one in which the knees are slightly bent, the weight is distributed over both feet and usually slightly forward. Initial body position will vary according to the situation, but appropriate adaptation of body position should be constantly evaluated and should allow the quickest and most effective response. Small excitatory rhythmical movements can be made which stimulate good muscular tension and open up the appropriate neural pathways. This form of preparation can be seen when receiving service in tennis or defending in volleyball.

Practice conditions should be similar to actual requirements, and there are a whole range of possible reaction-time practices for each individual sport. The following drills should provide a guide to the nature of the practice, models which can then be modified for the appropriate sport.

Reaction Drills

1. Work in pairs; partner A stands in ready position, partner stands behind A's back holding a tennis ball at head height. B drops the tennis ball and, on hearing the bounce on the floor, A turns to catch the ball before it bounces a second time. For progression, the difficulty can be increased by dropping the ball from shoulder height, hip height or knee height. It is effective to do a set number of repetitions at each height and produce a small schedule.

2. Work in pairs; partner B stands behind partner A on a line. With accurate feeding of height and distance to provide just the right challenge, B throws a tennis ball forward over A's shoulder; on first sight of the ball, A runs forward to make a catch before the second bounce.

3. Work in threes; B and C with a tennis ball each stand 5 metres apart; A faces B with a distance of 4 metres between them. B throws ball to A who returns it to B, then A runs to a point opposite C who throws it to A who returns it to C; A then runs back in front of B. This small pressure practice continues for a set time interval of 30 to 60 seconds.

These drills can be expanded and developed for the specificity of a sport. For example, a football can be rolled quickly to one side of a player who has to move rapidly to cut off the pass, then it is repeated on the other side.

Fast Feet

The aim is to move the feet as fast as possible. The steps taken are very small and the emphasis is on rapid movement. Keep tall and work the arms and shoulders. Speed ladders *(Fig 258)*, cones, hoops, tyres or similar markers can be used as equipment for these drills.

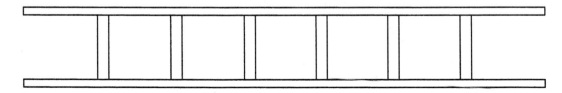

Fig 258 Speed ladder.

For example, move down the ladder, focusing on fast feet and very little knee lift:

1. Facing forward, place a foot in each slot.
2. Facing forward, place both feet one after the other in each slot.
3. Facing sideways, travel down the ladder placing both feet in each slot. Lead with right foot then change to lead with left foot.
4. Face ladder at the side and place one foot in the slots and the other below the ladder as you move along. Lead with left/right.
5. Face ladder at the side and place one foot in the slots; the other moves below and above the ladder as you move along. Alternate with leading left and right feet.

Other practices can be developed from these drills and the emphasis is always to move the feet as fast and as controlled as possible.

Quick Hands

Find a padded surface that can be hit such as a boxing bag, rugby tackle bag or martial arts/boxing focus gloves. Strike the target with the palm of your hand as many times as you can. Concentrate on performing firm and quick hits.

Running Speed

Running speed is determined by length and frequency of stride. Because the propulsive force is created by the extension of the driving leg (from which the other movements are derived), this factor should receive some attention when training for sprinting. The sprint training methods which follow need to be supplemented by carefully structured strength, power and flexibility work. Muscle groups such as the quadriceps, gluteals and gastrocnemius need to be strengthened to provide the capacity for the muscle to contract at a much faster rate. Co-ordination between the contracting (prime mover) and relaxing (antagonist) muscle groups will also improve with an appropriate strength and power training programme. Speed development will also be assisted by increased flexibility in the ankles, hips and shoulders.

Speed Drills

Many athletes train assiduously, sprinting impressive total distances but fail to become significantly faster and more efficient through poor form. Attention to the simple mechanics of sprinting will often produce gains in speed where strenuous work may do so only marginally. In addition to the sprint training some consideration should be given to good running form. The main aim of speed drills is to focus on key parts of the sprint action and attempt to control and refine them. The drills concentrate on the technique of running by working to achieve the efficient movement of arms and legs, about a still head and trunk. Elbows should be kept close to the body with a relaxed arm action working from the shoulders. The faster the speed, the more accentuated the arm action up and forward. Hands should be relaxed at all times and should not pass behind the hip joint.

Speed drills should be included regularly within the sprint training programme as the concentration on good technique forms the basis for all the other sprint training methods. During these drills emphasis is placed on maintaining techniques outlined. Two or three sets of each exercise can be used and intervals of rest will vary according to level of fitness.

1. Running on the spot. Partners face one another one metre apart and run on the spot in the following way; lifting the knees high, driving back the elbows, keeping the

shoulders square and looking straight at the partner. A small schedule can be introduced which requires running at speeds expressed as a fraction of the athlete's *maximum* speed:

a. Half-speed for 30 seconds with a 30 to 50 seconds' walk recovery.
b. Three-quarters speed for 20 seconds with a 30 to 50 seconds' walk recovery.
c. Seven-eighths speed for 15 seconds with a 30 to 50 seconds' walk recovery.

During these drills, emphasis is placed on maintaining technique. Two or three sets of each exercise can be used and intervals of rest will vary according to level of fitness.

Further drills can take place over a distance of 40–60m, alternating the drill with 'easy running' over 10m distances. The drills should be done on a running track or flat grass with the area clearly marked with cones. All effort should be in the region of 70 to 90 per cent.
2. High knees. Emphasis is on lifting the knee high and keeping it high for as long as possible, at the same time driving the elbows and shoulders during the movement and keeping 'tall', and keeping hips high and the body upright.
3. Heel kicking (flicks). Lift the heels from the floor up towards the buttocks and back to the floor as quickly as possible, at the same time driving the elbows and shoulders during the movement: keep the hips high and body upright.
4. High hops. Adopt a hopping action and drive up off each leg by raising the opposite knee. Work the elbows and shoulders keeping the hips high and body upright.
5. Elbow drive. Short runs accelerating over 20–30m, emphasizing the vigorous driving back of the elbow drive throughout the length of the run.

6. Driving practice. Short runs accelerating over 20 to 30m concentrating on driving away and trying to make contact with the ground as long as possible on each stride. The feeling is 'drive, drive, drive'. At the same time keep the muscles of the face and neck as loose and relaxed as possible.
7. Leaning drill. Stand on the line ready to accelerate over 20–30m. Keep the hands by the sides and lean forward. Keep leaning forward, keeping the body straight until you feel you will fall over. Then drive out over the 20–30m distance, concentrating on keeping the body straight and on accelerating as fast as possible. The initial steps should be small and the stride length will increase as the body comes up to the vertical. Concentrate on taking small steps and building the stride length over the 20–30m distance. Work on driving the elbows, arm positioning, 'Lip-to-Hip' and relaxed hands, wrists, neck and face.

During the drills, emphasis is placed on maintaining technique. Two or three sets of each exercise can be used, and intervals of rest will vary according to the level of fitness.

Sprint Training

Three basic types of speed can be identified:

1. acceleration;
2. pure speed;
3. speed endurance.

Acceleration

1. Repetition sprints from standing start: 10–30m. Walk back recoveries. One method of improving acceleration is to sprint against some form of resistance.
2. Find a gentle to medium slope about 15–40m in length. Sprint maximally up the hill. Walk gently back down.

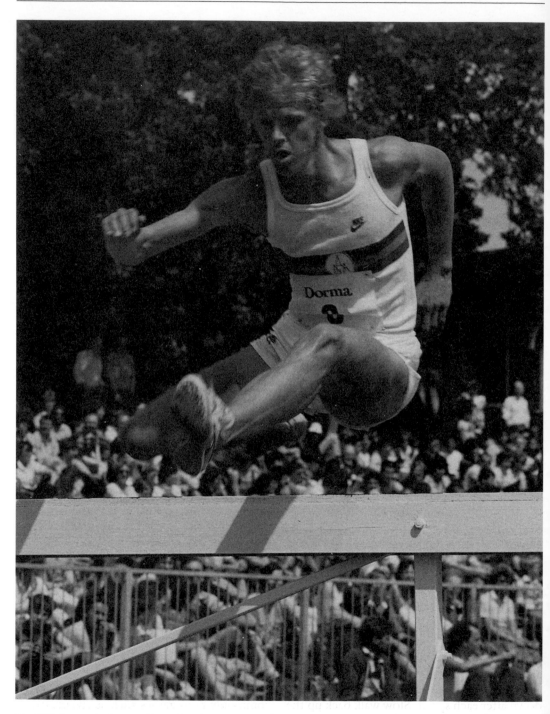

Fig 259 A steeplechase athlete showing power and endurance.

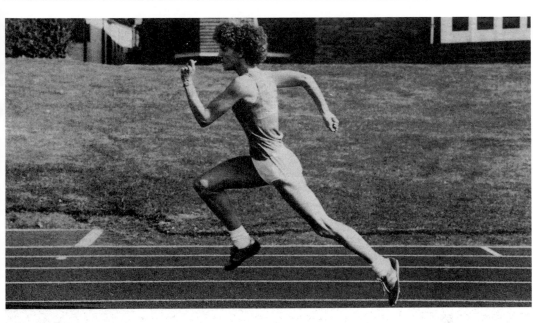

Fig 260 This sprinter shows good technique.

3. Harness running: use a two person harness which allows another person to provide the resistance. Attempt to sprint at 90 per cent of maximum speed.

4. Parachutes: parachutes of various sizes provide some degree of resistance.

Pure Speed

As with all other speed training, the effort level must be high, all efforts being close to, or at, full speed.

1. Six repetitions of 40–60m in sets of three to four. Slow walk back recoveries between repetitions with five minutes' rest between sets.

2. One way to increase speed is to let gravity help move your limbs a little quicker, so find a gentle downhill slope and sprint maximally downhill for 20–30m and gradually slow down after each sprint. Slow walk back up the slope; eight to ten repetitions.

3. Towing is another method of overspeed training and can produce higher stride rates and increase stride length. A 8m piece of elastic tubing is attached to the waist by a belt. The opposite end is attached to another athlete, or a stationary object such as a goalpost. Back up to stretch the tubing about 15–20m and run at three-quarters pace to adjust to the drill, then back up further until there is a distance of 35m, then sprint at high speed with the pull.

Ensure that all the necessary safety precautions and supervision are in place when using tubing and similar equipment for training.

Speed Endurance

In many sports athletes are required to sprint short distances, but there are occasional longer full-speed runs to perform and, more commonly as in games such as soccer, rugby and hockey, a series of such sprints are

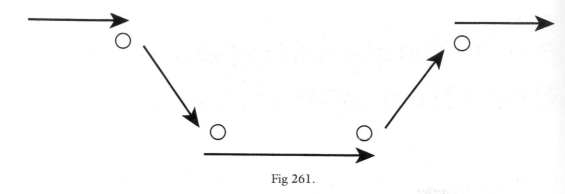

Fig 261.

required. This makes demands on an athlete's speed endurance in maintaining maximum speed over a period of time and recovering between a sequence of sprints in order to produce maximum effort during each sprint.

Training for speed endurance can involve four sets of five repetitions of 50m sprints at about 95 per cent effort with a 20 seconds' jog back recovery between repetitions and a two-minute rest between sets. An alternative session could be: Three sets of six repetitions of 60m at about 85 per cent effort with a 25-second jog back recovery between repetitions, and three-minute rest between sets.

Change of Pace and Direction

In addition to acceleration and pure running speed, many sports require athletes to be able to control and execute change of pace and direction, so it is important that speed training incorporates these factors.

Acceleration training involves a gradual increase from jogging, to half-pace, to striding out, to full pace. Markers need to be used so that the increase in pace occurs at particular points during the run. Rest interval is the walk-back recovery. Two to three sets of six sprints per set would be a recommended session.

Another practice for change of pace is hollow sprints which are two sprints interrupted by a period of recovery in the form of light running or jogging. You may accelerate 30–50m, jog 30–50m, accelerate again for 30–50m, then walk back the 100–150m as the recovery phase. Again, two to three sets of six sprints per set would be a typical session.

As with change of pace, in many sports athletes have to change direction whilst performing a sprint. Training for this could involve, for example, sprinting around a slalom course as shown in Fig 261.

The slalom course could be marked with poles, cones or similar markers. Perform three or four sets of ten repetitions with walk-back recoveries and two minutes' rest between sets.

Many different layouts and distances can be arranged to provide variety in training changes of direction and simulate situations in particular sports.

It can be seen that speed is a very wide-ranging factor and a particularly crucial one in many sports, especially at the higher levels of performance. Although genetic factors such as limb length and proportion of fast-twitch fibres do limit an athlete's maximum potential, everyone with the right training can improve their speed considerably.

CHAPTER 7
Body Composition, Nutrition and Diet

It is well appreciated in the fields of sports science, coaching and physical education that performance potential is determined to a large extent by hereditary factors. Each individual has a genetic potential, and height, physique and body composition will be of major importance in influencing achievement in a particular sport. While body shape or build can be altered only slightly, significant changes can be promoted in body composition which refers to the proportion of body fat and lean body weight. The latter term refers to all of the body tissue which is not fat, i.e. muscle, bone and organs. With athletes in training, any changes in weight will primarily result from changes in fat and muscle mass, so any changes in lean body weight will reflect changes in muscle mass. Total weight then may be considered as a composition of 'fat' weight and 'lean' weight.

BODY COMPOSITION

Body composition values tend to vary with different sports, but those which have a noticeable endurance factor will include athletes with low relative body fat. With the considerable range of body sizes and builds it is not possible to be too definitive, but it is true generally that an excess of body fat can be detrimental to performance in many activities. An excess of fat is dead weight that results in uneconomical effort. Speed is reduced, endurance diminishes and the likelihood of injury increases. As a general rule, the lower the relative body fat, the greater the performance potential of the athlete. So, rather than being concerned with overall weight most athletes should be particularly concerned with their lean body weight and relative changes in body fat.

There are a number of different techniques used but a measure of body fat percentage can be estimated by using anthropometric or body measurements. Numerous methods exist which measure different skinfold thicknesses (common sites include biceps, triceps, subscapular and suprailiac). These values are then plugged into equations and formulae which predict the percentage of the body weight which is fat. Taking measurements periodically has been shown to give special incentive to individual athletes needing to reduce their percentage of fat. Table 6 gives a general indication of the range of body fat percentages and their classification relative to athletic performance.

A large proportion of the population is concerned with weight control for one reason or another, so athletes are not unique in facing this challenge. The key to weight control is that caloric expenditure must match (or exceed) caloric intake; this is the basic notion of *energy balance*. By energy is meant the capacity to perform work. The concept of energy is a difficult one, but athletes are concerned mainly with two forms of energy. The human body converts

119

Table 6 Classification of per cent body fat for male and female athletes.

Sex	Body fat classification		
	Desirable	Acceptable	Over-fat
Male	8–12%	12–18%	18%+
Female	12–18%	18–26%	26%+

Per cent body fat categories are estimated from anthropometric measurements from male and female athletes aged 20–30 years

chemical energy, found in foodstuffs, into mechanical or *kinetic energy*. Mechanical work can be performed by acceleration of the body forwards (say) as in running, or the swinging of a cricket bat or tennis racquet performs mechanical work. Energy associated with movement is kinetic energy.

A calorie, the most common unit of measurement of energy is the amount of heat energy required to raise the temperature of one gram of water one degree Centigrade. Because foods contain a lot of energy, food energy is measured in kilocalories (kcal), which is equal to 1,000 calories, and is the unit most often used to describe the energy content of food and the energy requirements of the various physical activities.

More recently energy has been measured in joules (J). One joule is about 0.25 calories. One kilojoule is equal to 1,000 joules.

Losing Body Fat

From the basic concept of energy balance (intake of calories against calorie expenditure), the two processes which are of fundamental importance in weight control are losing body fat and gaining lean body mass. To lose body fat, a negative kilocaloric balance has to be achieved. The three possible ways of achieving this are to reduce the food intake, increase the exercise load, or a combination of both. If an athlete is training regularly, any reduction in percent body fat will be most directly linked to a reduced kilocaloric intake. The most efficient means of losing body fat is through a combined diet-exercise programme. It should be borne in mind that losing body fat requires long term planning and weight loss at a rate of one kilogram per week is usually recommended.

In terms of activity, long steady state (aerobic) exercise, i.e. running and cycling, is the optimal form of training for losing body fat. There is little evidence to support the notion of spot reducing of fat. Spot reducing refers to the exercise of a specific area of the body to achieve localized loss of fat. The general view is that fat is lost generally regardless of exercise selection.

Gain Lean Body Mass

Gaining lean body mass should be considered as a long term objective. In most cases a maximal rate gain in muscle mass is 0.5 to one kilogram per week from an appropriate training programme. Increasing muscle mass can only result from muscle overload supported by an adequate increase in food intake.

It is helpful to the athlete if body weight and percent body fat are monitored regularly to detect any unwanted increases in body fatness which would necessitate an increase in overload or, more likely, a reduction in food intake. The diet should have an optimal supply of all essential nutrients so that supplements are unnecessary, except in a specific case, for example when a female athlete may need an iron supplement. Contrary to general belief, the protein requirement for muscle growth is not greatly increased. A normal mixed diet will supply more than enough protein to build and repair muscles.

NUTRITION

One of the main aims of good nutrition for the athlete is to support training and performance. This means that the diet needs to provide sufficient energy for the demands of the training and the competitive programme. We often eat and drink without much thought and assume that our requirements will be met. We all enjoy eating and drinking socially and our choice of food is often based on 'eating for entertainment' rather than 'eating for energy'. However, the athlete in serious training has to ensure that his/her training demands are being met by his/her diet, and it is true to say that the diet can influence performance. As has been shown earlier, improvements in fitness are the result of the body adapting to the stress of training. The adaptations require the intake of necessary nutrients so the diet makes an impact during the recovery periods between training sessions when these adaptations are taking place.

Energy is derived mainly from the carbohydrate and fat in food and, to a lesser extent, protein. Once the carbohydrate is consumed it appears in the blood as glucose, which can then be used directly for energy or stored in the liver or muscle as glycogen, which is an important energy source for the athlete. A small amount can also be stored in the muscles.

The amount of energy stored as glycogen in the body is limited compared to the amount stored as fat. An athlete may have 14g of fat stored which, in energy terms, would allow him/her to run ten marathons one after the other!

During a training session and during competition, the muscles derive their energy from a combination of glycogen, (stored) carbohydrate and fat. The intensity and duration of the activity dictates the proportions of carbohydrate and fat used. If the training or competition is intensive and the energy is required rapidly, it is only the carbohydrates that can produce the energy fast enough. Only a small proportion of fat would be used at this level of effort.

Therefore, the harder the training or the effort during the competition, the more dependent the athlete is on the supply of carbohydrates the glycogen stores. To a certain extent, the amount of glycogen stored in the muscle (and the muscle can only use the glycogen which is stored within it – 'it cannot borrow from next door!') dictates the amount of work that can be done by that muscle. So one strong message about nutrition is that for an athlete in serious training and competition the diet should be high in carbohydrates with approximately 50 to 60 per cent of the total energy intake coming from that source. How is this achieved? Basically there are two main types of carbohydrates, complex and simple. When trying to increase the intake of carbohydrates emphasis should be placed on the former group, the complex carbohydrates: bread, potatoes, baked beans, cereals and fresh fruit such as bananas and dried fruit, prunes and apricots. Some reliance can be made on simple carbohydrates – sugars, confectionery or sweet foods – to add to the amount of carbohydrate required. To assist with the proportions of

121

carbohydrates (60 per cent) and fat (15 per cent) required, the overall amount of fat in the diet should be reduced.

Evidence on protein intake indicates that the normal dietary intake of about one gram of protein per kilogram of body weight is sufficient for athletes in training, including strength and power training programmes. A well-balanced, varied diet should meet the dietary demands of an athlete on a serious strength training programme. Increasing the amount of protein and consuming protein supplements is unlikely to have any beneficial effects. The message is very much for a high carbohydrate diet, which is in keeping with a healthy diet and will provide the best possible support to the athlete's training and performance in competition.

FLUID BALANCE

An important dietary factor for the athlete in training is fluid balance. Water is essential to life, although it is not strictly a nutrient. Water makes up about 60 per cent of a man's body and 50 per cent of a woman's. Among its many functions, it enables blood volume to be maintained; it provides a medium for all the complex biochemical reactions; it provides a medium for the transport and exchange of nutrients; and it assists in the regulation of body temperature. In non-active individuals about two litres of water is required per day to replace that lost and to maintain fluid balance, but this will not be sufficient for athletes in training who will lose a far greater amount of water. So fluid balance – hydration – is vital to the athlete in training as even a slight reduction in body water will reduce the efficiency in cellular function, and dehydration will deprive the body of sufficient water to cool itself and maintain body temperature within acceptable limits.

Thirst is an unreliable indicator of the need to start drinking fluids as the thirst mechanism is a delayed sign of the body's need for extra water. Firstly, it is important to maintain a high fluid intake as part of the normal diet, so drinking appropriate fluids on a regular basis, and then to be fully hydrated before training sessions, which means taking water about half an hour before training and then from time to time during the training session by taking appropriate 'fluid breaks'.

ORGANIZING THE DIET

Athletes are often busy people, having to organize their training and competition alongside many other commitments, so it is often the diet and nutrition which suffers within the whole training programme. It is important that the athlete organizes himself/ herself to eat sensibly and adequately in order to 'refuel' between training sessions and competitions. It is advisable, for example, to eat or drink carbohydrates directly after training sessions as there is evidence to show that the carbohydrate is absorbed more readily during this period. As it is advisable to eat regularly, an athlete may need to prepare snacks so that amounts of food can be consumed within a busy schedule. Rest days are an important part of the training programme as they allow the body to recover from the stresses of the training and for the adaptations to take place. So this is a key time to eat sensibly and refuel the carbohydrate stores.

The essential factor in the days leading up to the competition is to ensure that the 'fuel tank' is full. The ability of an athlete to perform high-intensity work is related to the initial glycogen stores in the muscles. How you have eaten in the days prior to the competition can influence your performance in terms of availability of energy required. So an adequate intake of carbohydrate is a necessity in the lead-up to competition. There should be a gradual increase in carbohydrate and fluid, particularly during the last two days, but do not overeat. Eat smaller, more frequent, high carbohydrate meals.

Day of Competition

Any meal on the day of competition should be light, easily digestible and be high in carbohydrate. It should be eaten three to four hours before the start of competition so there is adequate time for digestion, which means that the body's blood supply can concentrate on providing energy to the muscles and is not competing with blood flow to the digestive system. Also, anxiety experienced before competition will tend to slow down the rate of digestion.

Based on these guidelines, it is a matter of establishing what works best for the individual to fix a procedure of eating a certain meal which is part of the regular preparation process so that the athlete feels comfortable and familiar with the build-up to competition.

The influence of diet and nutrition on training and performance has been emphasized and, although occasional indulges in diet are of little consequence, the key thing is for the athlete to eat appropriately and sensibly 365 days of the year. This approach should effectively absorb the immediate dietary requirements of competition.

DIET

Everybody should follow a balanced diet. In the past, the main dietary problem was one of lack of vital nutrients; it was essential to ensure that everyone got enough protein, vitamins and minerals to keep healthy. Nowadays, if a person feels well and is neither too fat nor too thin, then his/her nutrition is probably satisfactory.

However, today there is a nutritional problem of a different kind, in that there is the danger of consuming too much of certain types of food and so putting a strain on some important body mechanisms. This can result in diet-linked disorders like obesity, anaemia, tooth decay, constipation and related bowel diseases, high blood pressure and heart disease. The following recommendations (generally accepted by medical experts) will help to offset the development of these disorders and provide the basis for healthy eating:

1. Absorb less sugar.
2. Consume less fat, especially animal fat.
3. Reduce intake of salt.
4. Reduce intake of alcohol.
5. Eat more dietary fibre.

Sugar

The average person absorbs over 45kg of sugar each year, not just in beverages and sprinkled over cereals but also in cakes, biscuits, puddings, tinned fruit, confectionery and drinks, in honey, jams and marmalade; and, more surprisingly, in canned and packet soups, baked beans and canned minced beef. Ideally, the average intake of sugar should be limited to 20kg of sugar each year which works out at about eleven level teaspoons a day, including the hidden sugar in other foods. Sugar is an empty food; it only provides energy. Other energy-giving foods like bread and potatoes provide not only energy but other valuable nutrients such as protein, vitamins and minerals.

To reduce sugar intake: gradually decrease, then cut sugar out of beverages; control a natural liking for sweet foods by eating an apple instead of a bar of chocolate for a snack; reduce sugar levels in recipes and eliminate puddings at the end of meals except for weekends, eating fruit instead.

Fat

Too much fat in the diet (if it is of animal origin) can lead to obesity and heart disease. Obvious fatty foods include butter, margarine, lard, dripping, cooking fats and oils, fat on meat and fried foods. Less obvious fatty foods include pastry, cakes, biscuits, chocolate, sauces, salad creams, mayonnaise, nuts, milk, cream, cheese, bacon, ham and sausages.

Fat adds flavour to food, and a certain amount is necessary as part of a balanced diet, but the first priority is to reduce the consumption of fat and then to replace animal fats (solid, hard, saturated fats) with vegetable fats and oils (soft or liquid polyunsaturated fats) whenever possible. The only true polyunsaturated oils are corn oil, soya bean oil, sunflower, safflower and cotton oils.

To reduce the intake of fat: avoid fatty meat and choose lean meat (although even this will have some hidden fat), chicken with skin removed, and white fish. Grill food rather than fry, placing the food on a wire rack so that all excess fat drains away, and fish and poultry in foil so that they can cook in their own juices. If food must be fried, use an oil low in saturated fat, i.e. a vegetable based oil whenever possible; and dry-fry minced beef to draw off the fat and discard it before adding vegetables and other ingredients. Do not spread margarine (preferably sunflower) or butter thickly on toast or bread. Use skimmed or semi-skimmed milk and choose low-fat cheeses.

Salt

The average intake of salt per person each day should not exceed 9g (just less than two teaspoons) including the hidden salt in food consumed. To reduce the daily intake of salt, try to control the use of salt by tasting the food first. Avoid the use of stock cubes and reduce salt to the absolute minimum when cooking. Herbs, spices and lemon juice all add flavour to dishes.

Alcohol

Alcohol, when digested, becomes an energy-giving food; in other words, if it is not burned up in exercise, it will be stored as fat. Because of this and other risk factors associated with alcohol consumption it is recommended that intake follows the well-publicized safe limits. Weight-for-weight, alcohol has more calories than protein or carbohydrate, with none of the nutritional value.

Fibre

Dietary fibre or 'roughage' is that part of the food not digested or absorbed by the body, but passed out as waste. It is a bulky substance and very absorbent. It is because of this particular property that its presence in the bowel is invaluable in ensuring that the bowel contents remain soft and thus are more easily eliminated from the body. In this way, it prevents constipation and there is a theory that it soaks up residual poisons from the tract, thus eliminating them regularly before they can cause harm. Foods rich in fibre include bran in cereals, wholemeal flour and bread, wholegrain cereals including whole wheat cereals, brown rice, brown pasta, peas and beans of all kind, lentils, root vegetables such as carrots, turnips and potatoes (eaten with the skin as jacket potatoes), dried fruits such as figs, raisins, dates, etc., and nuts, and all other fruits and vegetables.

Ways to Increase Fibre in the Diet

1. Choose wholemeal bread whenever possible, or at least brown bread.
2. Switch to wholemeal flour for all baking or bread, scones, pizzas, pastry and biscuits.
3. Choose a breakfast cereal that states 'bran'

or 'wholemeal' on the packet.

4. Buy brown unpolished rice, spaghetti and pasta; these take longer to cook but are more filling and nutritious than their refined counterparts.

5. Add plenty of beans, peas and lentils to soup, casseroles, curries and salads.

6. Eat plenty of root vegetables, especially potatoes baked in their skins.

7. Leave skins on fruits like apples, pears and peaches.

MEAL IDEAS FOR ATHLETES
(with emphasis on a high carbohydrate/low fat diet)

Ideas for Breakfast

- Skimmed or semi-skimmed milk, low fat spread and wholemeal bread are ideal choices. Sugar added to cereals is an individual choice.
- Any of the following cereals with skimmed or semi-skimmed milk and sugar if desired: Cornflakes; one or two Weetabix; Branflakes; Shredded Wheat, Fruit and Fibre.
- Additions to the above: sliced or chopped banana, sultanas, raisins, chopped dried fruit, e.g. peaches, apricots.
- Porridge or Ready Brek, with milk and golden syrup or sugar.
- One glass of any unsweetened fruit juice.
- Half a fresh grapefruit or any fresh fruit, e.g. apples, pears, oranges, grapes, melon.
- Tinned grapefruit in natural juice.
- Diet yoghurt mixed with oats, sultanas and chopped banana.
- Two bananas or melon, chopped and added to a diet yoghurt.
- Lean grilled bacon with grilled tomato halves (or tinned tomatoes), boiled or scrambled egg (cooked fatless in non-stick pan or microwaved), mushrooms microwaved with no fat.

- Baked beans, tinned tomatoes.
- Wholemeal bread or crusty bread roll with low-fat spread and jam, marmalade, honey or Marmite.

Ideas for Packed Lunches

Wholemeal bread or rolls, French bread, pitta bread or wholegrain Ryvita (but have fillings separately) and low-fat spread if required with:

- Hard-boiled egg with low-fat mayonnaise.
- Lean ham, beef, pork, chicken, turkey.
- Low-fat cottage cheese.
- Tuna (canned in water or brine).
- Salmon, prawns, (fresh or canned), sardines, pilchards.
- Mustard, pickle, low-fat mayonnaise or salad cream, beetroot, gherkins, tomato ketchup.
- Lettuce, watercress, white cabbage, red onion, spring onions, cucumber, tomatoes.
- To eat with sandwiches: carrot and celery sticks, cherry tomatoes, beansprouts, red onion rings, spring onions, slices of red, green and yellow peppers, bean, rice and pasta salads with low-fat dressings.

Ideas for Lunches

- Jacket potatoes topped with any of the following: baked beans, sweetcorn, low-fat cottage cheese, tuna (in brine or water), chopped chicken pieces and sweetcorn in plain yoghurt with half-teaspoon of curry powder, coleslaw, shredded white cabbage, grated carrot with low-fat mayonnaise.
- Toasted sandwiches with salad, e.g. ham and tomato sandwich toasted and served with a tossed salad or cheese and thinly sliced onion.
- Cup-a-soup (low-fat variety).
- With toast: plain or curried baked beans, tinned spaghetti, ravioli, tomatoes or

microwaved fresh tomatoes, scrambled egg (in microwave), poached egg, sardines (in tomato sauce).

Ideas for Dinners

As a general rule, foods with a very high fat content should be avoided, such as cream, sausages, cheap beefburgers, salami, patc, cheese (except for low-fat varieties like Edam, Shape, Tendale, etc.), crisps and all similar savoury snacks, nuts, battered foods and other food that has been fried.

Grilling and microwaving are the recommended methods for cooking meat and fish, but roasting bags to use in conventional and microwave ovens are excellent and are available from all supermarkets.

Potatoes can be boiled, mashed, baked or microwaved. It is possible to dry-roast potatoes by boiling even-sized pieces in salted water for five minutes, draining well, placing on a non-stick baking tray and baking for about one hour on Gas Mark 6–7, 210–220°C.

All other accompanying vegetables can be cooked in the usual ways, whether fresh of frozen.

- Chicken or turkey cooked in the oven using a roasting bag (see above), eaten with the skin removed. Gravy made using low-fat gravy powder.
- Grilled gammon steaks with pineapple rings (in natural juice).
- Grilled white fish with tomato sauce – a tin of chopped tomatoes reduced until thick, mixed with two tablespoons of tomato puree, Worcester sauce, salt and pepper. Frozen peas may be added at the end, cooked in the mixture.
- Shepherd's pie can be made using soya savoury mince which is totally fat-free.
- Spaghetti Bolognese – using lean minced beef.

- Grilled beef steak – dry-fried or grilled; sliced onions can be microwaved.
- Cheese and vegetable bake: boil a selection of vegetables for about 10 to 15 minutes: thickly sliced new potatoes, carrots, onions and leeks, adding cauliflower, broccoli florets for the last five minutes; drain and add sliced mushrooms. Put into an ovenproof dish, cover with cheese sauce, sprinkle the top with grated cheese and bake for about one hour at Gas Mark 4, 180°C until golden and the vegetables are completely cooked.
- Tuna and pasta bake – similar to the above. Boiled pasta shells and flaked tuna mixed with cheese sauce and vegetables baked for about 30 minutes at Gas Mark 4, 180°C.
- Chicken, prawn or vegetable chop suey. This is a stir-fry without fat. The chicken is cooked slowly in about one tablespoon of vegetable stock, then vegetables are added and stir-fried in the juices until cooked. Serve with brown rice and soya sauce.

Ideas for Puddings

- All fresh and stewed fruit with diet custard (carton) or diet yoghurt or fromage frais.
- Chopped melon added to any flavour of diet yoghurt.
- Cream pears – halved, peeled and cored ripe pears filled with fromage frais; if plain fromage frais, add apricot jam.
- Meringue nest filled with fresh fruit, raspberry, strawberry, or banana and topped with diet yoghurt or fromage frais.
- Baked stuffed apple – slit a baking apple skin around the middle, core and fill the cavity with sultanas and brown sugar. Microwave for about two minutes and serve with a carton of diet custard.
- Fresh fruit salad and diet yoghurt or fromage frais.

CHAPTER 8
Fitness Testing

Fitness tests can be administered at various stages during the training programme to measure and monitor progress, and evaluate the effects of the training. The results of these tests provide a 'fitness profile' of the athlete, identifying strengths and weaknesses that can be used in the future planning of the fitness training. This allows for the more individual training programme on the particular needs of the athlete. Therefore, they should always be seen as a means to an end – a way of monitoring progress linked with the planning of the programme.

There are a number of fitness components that can be measured, for example;

- Aerobic endurance
- Muscular endurance
- Upper body strength
- Leg power
- Flexibility
- Speed and acceleration
- Anaerobic capacity
- Body composition.

AEROBIC ENDURANCE

Simple field tests of endurance can be devised to evaluate improvements in aerobic fitness. Depending on the condition of the athlete, distances of one, two and three kilometres can be used for a timed run, preferably on an athletics track or on a games field with a known measured distance.

A useful indicator of an athlete's endurance fitness is the measurement of 'maximum oxygen uptake'. The symbol is $\dot{V}O_2max$. This is the greatest amount of oxygen that an athlete can take from the air and transport via the lungs, heart and circulation to the working muscles. This is the basic form of fitness – the capacity to keep working and delay the onset of fatigue over a prolonged period of time. In many sports the athlete has to perform over a prolonged period, so this is a vital fitness quality.

Maximum oxygen uptake ($\dot{V}O_2max$) is frequently measured in sports science laboratories using treadmill or bicycle ergonometer. This testing facility is not available to many athletes, so the use of field testing can be more appropriate.

There are a number of field tests which provide an indirect determination of maximum oxygen uptake ($\dot{V}O_2max$). One effective test which is fairly easy to administer uses a 20km shuttle run. The test requires the athlete to run 20m at a pace dictated by a sound signal emitted from a cassette recorder. Each minute the pace of the shuttle is increased. The athlete has to keep pace with the sound signal for as long as possible. The point at which the athlete can no longer keep up with the dictated pace is recorded and used to estimate $\dot{V}O_2max$. For example, if an athlete reaches level 11 he/she will have a predicted $\dot{V}O_2max$ of 50.4 ml/kg × min. Multi-Stage Fitness tapes are available from the National Coaching Foundation in Leeds.

Table 7 Estimated V̇O₂max for 1½ mile run time.

Time (min. sec)	Estimated V̇O₂max (ml/kg × min)	Classification (aerobic fitness)
7.30 and under	75	
7.31–8.00	72	
8.01–8.30	67	HIGH
8.31–9.00	62	
9.01–9.30	58	
9.31–10.00	55	GOOD
10.01–10.30	49	
10.31–11.00	46	AVERAGE
11.01–11.30	44	
11.31–12.00	41	
12.01–12.30	39	
12.31–13.00	37	FAIR
13.01–13.30	36	
13.31–14.00	33	
14.01–14.30	31	
14.31–15.00	30	LOW

Adapted from K.H. Cooper, 'A means of assessing maximum oxygen uptake', *Journal of the American Medical Association*, **203**, 201–204, 1968. The range of V̇O₂max values will vary with age and sex. The classification is based on a population of males aged 20–29 years. Estimated values for females of this age range can be obtained by moving up one category. Adapted from J.H. Wilmore, *Athletic Training and Physical Fitness*, Boston, Mass, Allyn and Bacon, 1976.

A long-established test is the Balke 1½-mile run. This is timed, and an estimated relationship between the time taken to complete the distance and V̇O₂max is provided with a simple classification of aerobic fitness (*see* Table 7).

MUSCULAR ENDURANCE

Push-ups *(Fig 262)*

Athletes perform an extended push-up that measures the muscle groups of the arms, shoulders and chest. To adopt the correct position the athlete lies on the mat in a prone position with arms out to the sides and elbows flexed at 90 degrees. The hands are then placed where the elbows were positioned. The test starts with the arms extended and feet together. The athlete then lowers by flexing the arms until the chest touches a tester's closed fist, placed on a mat immediately under the chest. He/she then pushes upwards to extend the arms, and then does as many push-ups as possible until he/she loses form by not being able to touch the fist with the chest, not extending the arms fully or not being able to maintain the repetitions. This test can also be performed to a controlled series of bleeps on an audio-cassette, for example, at 50 beats per minute.

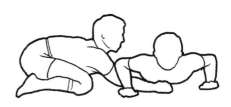

Fig 262.

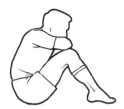

Fig 263.

Abdominals *(Fig 263)*

The athlete performs a trunk curl which measures a form of abdominal fitness. The athlete lies on his/her back with bent legs, feet flat on the floor unsupported and arms folded across the chest with hands on opposite shoulders, then rises to touch the thighs with the elbows and then lowers to touch the shoulders to the floor. The athlete does as many trunk curls as possible until he/she loses form by not touching the thighs with the elbows, by moving hands from the shoulders or not being able to maintain the repetitions. This test can also be performed to a controlled series of bleeps on an audio-cassette, for example at 50 beats per minute; or alternatively an Abdominal Fitness Tape is available from the National Coaching Foundation.

UPPER BODY STRENGTH

Because of the varied strength and power qualities required in sport, a range of strength tests can be used. To measure absolute strength – the maximum force that a muscle can exert against a resistance – the one repetition maximum (1RM) on a selected exercise can be measured. A whole range of exercises can be used so one example for this type of test is bench press (*see* Chapter 5, page 91, for technique), or an exercise machine can be similarly used. The athlete is given a number of attempts at increasing resistances until the maximum weight that he/she can lift *once* is established (1RM). Alternatively it can be the maximum weight that can be lifted twice (2RM) or three times (3RM). This approach can be used for a number of muscle groups. A variation of this test is to use a percentage of an athlete's body weight, for example 80, 90, or 100 per cent, and he/she would be asked to perform as many repetitions of the bench press as possible against a selected percentage of body weight.

STATIC STRENGTH

Lateral Hang *(Fig 264)*

Set a beam or bar so that you can hang with feet clear of the floor. Take an overgrasp hold on beam, pull up so that the eyes are above the top line of the beam. Hold the position for as long as possible; take the time from when you are looking over the beam until you drop from that position. You should neither touch the beam nor rest any part of your head on it; nor kick, struggle or move the body. One attempt only.

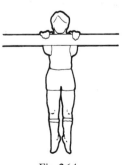

Fig 264.

ARM AND SHOULDER POWER

Medicine Ball Throw *(Fig 265)*

Lie on back with arms behind head holding a medicine ball. By pulling forward with the arms only and the back flat to the floor throw the medicine ball over the feet as far as possible. Measure distance from starting position of medicine ball to where it lands. Best of three attempts.

LEG POWER

Sargent Jump *(Fig 266)*

A board with horizontal lines marked in centimetres is fixed to a wall with the base just below stretch height. Stand next to wall and reach up with one arm to place hand on measuring board; note height. By bending and explosively extending the knees execute a vertical jump swinging the arms up and touching the measuring board with one hand; note height at top of fingers. Measure between the two noted heights. Best of three attempts.

Standing Broad Jump *(Fig 267)*

Toes to a line, bend at knees, swing arms and spring forward from both feet. The nearest point touched by any part of the body, at right angles to the take-off line is the distance to be measured. Best of three attempts.

Jump Meter *(Fig 268)*

Possibly a more accurate alternative to the Sargent Jump test is the use of a jump meter. The meter is fixed around the waist of the athlete with the end of the cord attached to a rubber mat on which the athlete stands. The athlete bends at the knees and drives vertically upwards

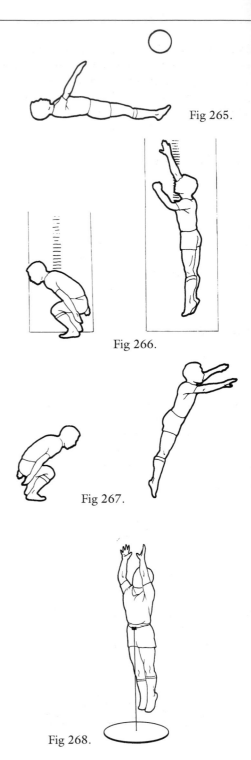

Fig 265.

Fig 266.

Fig 267.

Fig 268.

from the mat. The height of the vertical jump is recorded on the meter. There are now more advanced pieces of equipment which assess leg power by measuring the length of time an athlete lifts his/her body off the floor.

FLEXIBILITY

Flexibility can be measured indirectly or directly. The following are examples of simple indirect tests which can be affected by factors such as limb length, but these tests are designed not to judge one athlete against another, rather to measure your own progress so that your improvement can be objectively observed.

Indirectly

Sit and Reach (Fig 269)

The legs are kept straight, toes pointing vertically upward, head held up and fingers touching the toes. Measure distance from finger tips to toes – it could be a plus or minus score. If the finger tips extend beyond the toes, it is a plus score, if they cannot, it is a minus score.

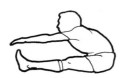

Fig 269.

Forward Flexion (Fig 270)

Sit with legs spread apart and straight, forearms on the floor, one fist on top of the other fist. Measure distance from forehead to top of

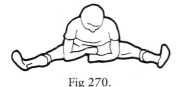

Fig 270.

fists. If the forehead can pass below the fists, it is a plus score, if it cannot, it is a minus score.

Shoulder Extension (Fig 271)

One arm is placed over the shoulder, the other behind the back. Move both hands towards one another and attempt to touch finger tips. If the finger tips overlap, it is a plus score, if they do not meet, it is a minus score.

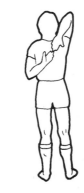

Fig 271.

Upward-Backward Movement of Arms (Fig 272)

Lie in a prone position with the chin touching the floor, and the arms reaching forward directly in front of the shoulders. Hold a rod or staff horizontally with both hands. Keep the elbows and wrists straight and chin on the floor, then raise the arms upward as far as possible. The score is the vertical distance from the floor to the lower side of the rod.

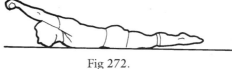

Fig 272.

Sideward-Backward Movement of Arms (Fig 273)

Stand with back against a wall, and raise arms to the horizontal with the palms forward. Keeping the arms horizontal and the fifth finger of each

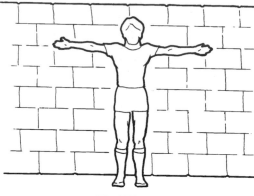

Fig 273.

hand in contact with the wall, move forward away from the wall as far as possible. Measure the horizontal distance from the wall to the spine at arm level.

Trunk Extension (Fig 274)

Lie on floor with hands clasped behind back (near small of back). With a partner pressing downward on the back of the legs, lift the chest off the floor as high as possible. Measure the distance from the supra-sternal notch to the floor.

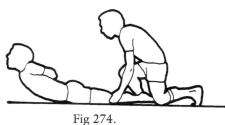

Fig 274.

Directly

Hip Flexion (Fig 275)

Direct assessments of flexibility measure the angle itself and they can provide a truer reflection of the extent of any improvement in the range of movement at a joint. There are a range of direct flexibility tests, but one useful example measures hip flexion.

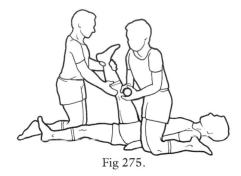

Fig 275.

A goniometer can be used and passive measurements will be made where the limb is moved into position by the tester and the athlete is asked to be as relaxed as possible. As with all tests which measure the limbs, both sides of the body are assessed to check for imbalances.

The athlete lies on his/her back with both legs straight. Two testers are required. Tester 1 kneels on the right side of the athlete and places his/her left hand on the ankle of the athlete. With his/her right hand, Tester 1 lifts the athlete's left leg until he/she feels a mild tension. Both legs are kept straight during the measurement. Tester 2 kneels on the left side of the athlete, places a goniometer against the athlete's left knee and reads off the measurement in degrees from the goniometer. Exactly the same procedure is used for the right leg.

SPEED AND ACCELERATION
(Fig 276)

The standard method of measuring running speed is to time the athlete over selected distances. This is acceptable, but there are problems associated with accurate timing, particularly over shorter distances when using a stopwatch, because of human error and false starts. Also, the improvement in sprinting times will be small and the testing needs to be

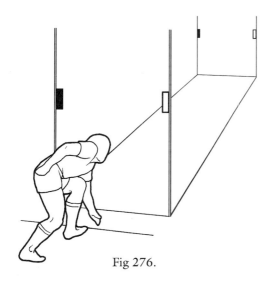

Fig 276.

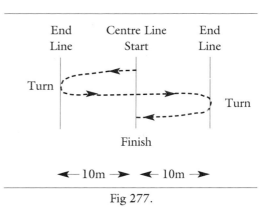

Fig 277.

sensitive enough to record accurately the small increases which occur. It is, therefore, more effective, if it can be afforded, to use electronic timing with photo-electric cells. The athlete stands one metre behind the first beam and timing will begin once the first beam has been broken and will be stopped when the athlete crosses the beam of the finish line.

In between, with the necessary equipment, many arrangements can be used: a range of distances, for example from 5–50m; testing at 5m or 10m stages; allowing the athlete to achieve top speed and then testing between two beams; or providing a course with changes of direction in between the start and finish of the sprint.

ANAEROBIC CAPACITY

This measures an athlete's capacity to produce a high level of effort for a short period of time and keep producing fast sprints or short bouts of high intensity work. The test provides an estimation of speed endurance based on a fatigue index. The athlete is required to sprint at a maximum speed over a 40m shuttle with a 20 seconds' recovery period between the sprints. The time for each shuttle sprint is recorded using a stopwatch.

Test Procedure *(Fig 277)*

1. The athlete starts with his/her feet behind the centre line.
2. He/she sprints to the end line (10m), turns and sprints to the far end line (20m), turns and sprints to the centre line (10m): total 40m.
3. Maximal effort is required for all sprints: no pacing.

Fatigue Index

A fatigue index, used to assess an athlete's speed endurance, is calculated by taking the average of his/her two fastest sprints away from the average of the two slowest sprints. The time difference between the two fastest and the two slowest sprints is then expressed as a percentage of the two fastest sprints. The percentage decrease in time between the two fastest and the two slowest sprints can be expressed by this formula:

$$(T7 + T8/2) - (T1 + T2/2) = D$$
$$D/(T1 + T2/2) \times 100 = X\%$$

Table 8 Example calculation of fatigue index.

	Sprint	
1	8.66	(1) Mean of two slowest times minus mean of two fastest times:
2.	8.59	
3.	8.74	
4.	8.73	(2) Difference between fastest and slowest divided by the mean of
5.	8.70	the two fastest as a percentage:
6.	8.98	
7.	8.88	
8.	8.95	

$$\frac{8.98 + 8.95}{2} - \frac{8.66 + 8.59}{2} = 0.34$$

$$\frac{0.34 \times 100}{8.62} = 3.94\%$$

Fatigue index = 3.9%

where:

T1 and T2 = the two fastest sprints;

T7 and T8 = the two slowest sprints;

D = Difference;

X% = % drop in pace.

It may be simpler to calculate the fatigue index by subtracting the fastest time recorded from the slowest time, that is, 9.1 seconds (slowest) – 8.1 (fastest) = 1.0 (fatigue factor).

BODY COMPOSITION

In simple terms the human body may be regarded as being composed of two 'compartments', lean body mass (muscle, bones and organs), and body fat. Together they make up the total body weight. For an athlete in training the proportion of body fat to lean body mass (the body composition) can be more important to monitor than actual body weight. As a result of training an increase in muscle mass (making up lean body mass) may be accompanied by a decrease in body fat resulting in little change in total body weight. Also, an increase in body weight may occur if the increase in muscle mass exceeds the loss in body fat. So overall body weight may not be that informative for the athlete in training, so in addition to measuring weight and height it can be useful to monitor the body composition of an athlete. Methods of electronic fat measurement are available, but they may vary in reliability.

The weight of an athlete is taken, followed by measuring the skinfold thickness at four sites on the body: triceps, biceps, subscapular and suprailiac. The measurements are used in conjunction with approved methods and tables which are available for the estimation of body fat and lean body mass. On average, body fat accounts for 15 per cent of the total body weight for males and 25 per cent for females, but these figures are normally lower for male and female athletes actively involved in fitness training and competitive sport.

Standard measurements of weight and height can be taken for each athlete. Skinfold thickness can be measured at four sites on the body (triceps, biceps, subscapular and the iliac crest) and used in conjunction with approved methods for the calculation and estimation of body fat and lean body mass (Fig 278).

Skinfold thicknesses are measured on:

• triceps – with the arm hanging vertically relaxed, midway between the tip of the acromion process and the olecranon process
• biceps – with the arm resting supinated,

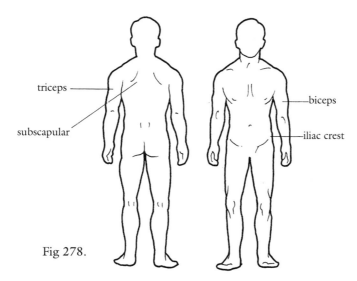

triceps

subscapular

biceps

iliac crest

Fig 278.

over the belly of the muscle, at the same level as the triceps

- subscapular – under the inferior angle of the scapula, the fold pointing slightly downwards and outwards
- iliac crest – 1cm above the iliac crest at the sides of the body with the fold running forwards and downwards.

The skinfold is picked up between thumb and forefinger and pulled slightly away from the underlying tissues. The calliper jaws are applied immediately below the finger and thumb. The measurement should be read on the callipers after the full pressure of the jaws has been applied which is two seconds after release of the trigger (Fig 279).

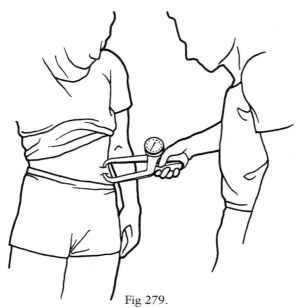

Fig 279.

CHAPTER 9
Rest, Recovery and Relaxation

Athletes naturally tend to concentrate their attention on the actual training, completing their various schedules in the bid for increased fitness; but this needs to be balanced with adequate rest, recovery and relaxation. An athlete should consider *in total* the factors that will influence the effects of training and increases in fitness. This encompasses the training programme, good nutrition and adequate rest and recovery.

REST AND RECOVERY

Rest should be seen as an integral part of the training programme. In the Introduction to Training (Chapter 2) it was shown that adaptations take place in the period following training leading to improvements in fitness, so it is important to rest adequately to allow this process to happen. It was also shown that in the cycle of training there is a recuperation phase, which is necessary to help athletes recover from the demands of a hard competitive season.

It is also necessary to help the body to recover from training sessions and competitions. This begins with an adequate cool-down, which was explained in Chapter 1. To achieve an effective recovery from a hard bout of competition, in the days following it is advisable to do some recovery sessions of light exercise (perhaps non-weight bearing), for example swimming or cycling. This increases blood flow through the muscles and around the body, which helps to remove waste products and supply oxygen, both of which aid recovery. This will also help with any muscle soreness. Also it is advisable to maintain flexibility during this period. In addition to recovery sessions of light exercise, massage has also been shown to help the recovery process and provide a degree of relaxation. The advice on fluid intake and diet in Chapter 7 is relevant for an adequate recovery. Keep well hydrated by drinking appropriate fluids during this period and try to eat soon after competition, a little and often is best (about 50g of carbohydrate per hour). An important contributor to rest and recovery is the amount and quality of sleep – as a guide, take at least eight hours each night.

RELAXATION

Rest and relaxation are naturally closely related. Relaxation can promote sleep by the elimination of tensions and thoughts that may result from an imminent competition or a particularly intensive phase of training.

Relaxation is the opposite of movement. It is characterized by a reduction of activity in the muscles which is accompanied by a lowering of activity in the rest of the body with heart rate, respiratory rate and other regulatory functions working at a lower pace. Relaxation is a neuromuscular function which results in a lowering of tension in the skeletal muscles; in other words, minimal muscular activity.

Relaxation is a skill which an athlete can learn. The area of relaxation is complex with all the psychosomatic implications, so it is only possible to provide a brief outline to ensure a balanced and complete approach is adopted in the pursuit of fitness. Relaxation techniques can be used to lower general muscular tension. This is particularly applicable during competition in any breaks between events or matches, or in rest intervals between hard bouts of training. Relaxation is also important during the build-up phase immediately prior to competition, to allow the athlete to achieve the right level of arousal and controlled mental preparation.

Relaxation Techniques

A relaxation technique suitable for athletes is *neuromuscular relaxation* in which the aim is to develop in the muscles a sensitivity to different levels of tension. The important message is that relaxation techniques have to be learned and practised in the same way that any sport's skill has to be learned. Neuromuscular relaxation, or *progressive relaxation* as it is called, was developed by Jacobson many years ago. The technique is learned by developing as much tension as possible in a particular muscle group, then relaxing to release the tension. It is progressive in that the athlete moves from one muscle group to another, and the learning factor is recognizing the level of tension in the muscle so attention is focused on the muscle and the tension being developed. The aim is to train this sensitivity to tension in the muscle. The full range of the technique needs to be learned correctly, but a brief example should give an indication of the approach.

As relaxation is the key factor, the session can take place after some training in which the exercising itself will tend to reduce tension. Also, it is useful to learn to relax after exercise. You should get into a comfortable position, preferably lying on your back, fully relaxed. Hips and legs are relaxed in such a way that the feet flop out to the side a little, arms are alongside the body, with elbows slightly flexed. The position should allow all muscle groups to be relaxed, and it may be necessary to have some form of support underneath the neck and knees.

Flex the right foot, trying to push the toes against the front of the leg; hold this position, then quickly let go and relax; repeat this a few times. Now do this with half that tension and repeat. Then again with even less tension. Try to develop an awareness of levels of tension.

An entire sequence is then done with the other foot. A series of similar exercises can then be done by pointing the toes and extending the ankle joints. Sequences can be repeated with the legs slightly raised off the floor and conversely with feet and legs pressed hard into the floor. The idea is to contract muscles, then relax and recognize the difference between tension and relaxation in the muscle. Then try different degrees of tension: half, quarter, minimal. The athlete then progresses from one muscle group to the next; feet and legs, abdominals, back and buttocks, hands and arms, shoulders, neck and face.

Differential Relaxation

From the basis of progressive relaxation, which involves working through all muscle groups as comprehensively as time permits, the athlete could develop to *differential relaxation* where the aim is to relax all muscles except those working. This can be done in weight training, where the athlete being proficient in the techniques of relaxation, attempts to relax all the muscles not being used in a particular weight training exercise. The aim is relaxation on the one hand, and concentration of energy solely into the task being performed. With a good grounding in progressive relaxation techniques the athlete becomes sensitive to the degree of tension in all the muscle groups.

Meditation

Progressive relaxation concentrates on the degrees of tension in the muscles and the subsequent effect on the central nervous system and the brain. Most other relaxation techniques concentrate on mental control and the flow of information (efferent nerve supply) to the muscle. Examples of these techniques would be meditation, autogenic training and visualization.

Meditation is a mental technique using a mantra, a non-stimulating meaningless sound which provides a focus for attention in a very passive manner. Very simply it prevents a person's mind from wandering by passively focusing on the mantra. There is a reduction in nervous stimulation which produces a relaxing effect, but the practice of meditation is also a useful method of increasing concentration.

Autogenic Training

Autogenic training involves self-induced responses to develop a deep state of relaxation. The technique, one of auto-hypnosis or self hypnosis, uses a series of exercises to produce two physical sensations – warmth and heaviness. Attention is focused on producing these sensations, and the training involves several months or more of regular practice to become proficient enough to experience heaviness and warmth in the limbs, a sensation of relaxed calm heart and respiratory rates, accompanied by warmth in the abdominal region (which produces a calming effect on the central nervous system and enhances muscular relaxation) and coolness in the forehead. The method uses auto-suggestion as a means of training for relaxation, which is followed by training in autogenic meditation involving imagery or visualization. The full range of autogenic training takes a relatively long time, but it has proved effective with particular athletes.

Visualization

Visualization techniques are suitable for athletes who have the ability to visualize easily. It is a method of imagining oneself in an environment conducive to relaxation. The particular object of visualization will be personal, but obvious examples are lying on a secluded beach in the warm sunshine or walking in very scenic peaceful countryside. In another way, visualization can be used as mental preparation before competition, where the athlete visualizes himself/herself performing particular skills competently.

Relaxation techniques vary from simple mental exercises to extensive forms of training. Choice or use of a relaxation technique will vary considerably with the individual athlete and will require adequate study by obtaining literary or taped information, or by attending a recognized course of training.

BALANCE

The rationale for considering rest, recovery and relaxation as a component of fitness is in providing the right balance between the stress placed on the body through the different forms and intensities of exercise and training, and the body's need to rest and relax. This balance can be expressed in a number of ways in sport. Each athlete will have an optimal level of arousal to maximize performance in which relaxation will be used as a control. Any training programme has to find the most effective mix of rest and the amount of physical exertion prescribed. During competition, the athlete requires the right blend of relaxation which will enhance alertness and awareness together with positive concentration and aggressiveness. In many ways, giving attention to the rest, recovery and relaxation factors will assist the process of training and help significantly to realize potential in performance.

Glossary

Adenosine Diphosphate (ADP) Chemical compound that is the product of ATP breakdown.

Adenosine Triphosphate (ATP) High energy chemical compound which is formed with the energy released from food and is stored in all cells, particularly muscle cells. Used as energy supply for muscle and other body functions; the energy currency.

Adipose Tissue Tissue in which fat is stored.

Aerobic In the presence of oxygen; aerobic metabolism utilizes oxygen.

Anaerobic In the absence of oxygen; non-oxidative metabolism.

Antagonist Name given to a muscle or muscles which cause the opposite action from that of prime movers.

ATP–PC System An anaerobic energy system in which ATP is manufactured when phosphocreatine is broken down.

Blood Pressure The driving force which moves blood through the circulatory system. The force exerted against the walls of the arteries.

Calorie A unit of work or energy equal to the amount of heat required to raise the temperature of one gram of water one degree Centigrade.

Capillaries Small vessels in a fine network located between the arteries and veins where oxygen, food, hormones are delivered to tissues and carbon dioxide and waste products are picked up.

Carbohydrate A chemical compound containing carbon, hydrogen and oxygen. Carbohydrates are one of the basic foodstuffs which we use for energy, stored in muscle and liver as glycogen.

Cardiorespiratory Pertaining to the circulatory and respiratory systems.

Cardiovascular System The heart and blood vessels.

Central Nervous System The portion of the nervous system consisting of the brain and the spinal cord.

Chemical Energy Energy associated with chemical transformations.

Concentric Contraction Shortening of the muscle during a muscular contraction.

Creatine Phosphate A molecule that transfers phosphate and energy to ADP to generate ATP.

Eccentric Contraction Muscular contraction in which the muscle lengthens while developing tension.

Energy The capacity to do work.

Energy Balance The balance which results when calorific expenditure equals calorie intake.

Enzyme A protein compound which speeds up chemical reactions.

Extension Straightening movement resulting in an increase in the angle of the joint by moving bones apart.

Fat A foodstuff containing glycerol and fatty acids. An important energy source, stored for future use when excess fat, carbohydrate or protein is ingested.

Fatigue Diminished work capacity; a state of tiredness, discomfort and decreased efficiency resulting from prolonged or excessive exertion.

Flexion Movement of bones towards each other at a joint by decreasing the angle between them.

Glucose A form of sugar; an energy source transported in the blood.

Glycogen Storage form of glucose found in muscles and liver.

Glycolysis Breakdown of glycogen to lactic acid.

Heart Rate (HR) The number of times the heart beats in a minute.

Hypertrophy An increase in the size of a cell or organ.

Isokinetic Muscular contraction against a resistance which is varied to maintain high tension throughout the range of movement while speed remains constant.

Isometric Muscular contraction in which tension is developed but with no change in the length of the muscle; contraction against an immovable resistance.

Isotonic Muscular contraction in which the muscle alters its length with varying tension while working against resistance.

Joule Work done (or energy converted) in moving a force of one newton a distance of one metre (one newton is the force needed to accelerate a mass of one kilogram at a rate of one metre per second per second).

Kilocalorie A unit of work or energy equal to the amount of heat required to raise the temperature of one kilogram of water one degree Celsius.

Kilogram A metric unit of weight equal to 2.2 pounds.

Kinetics The forces associated with the movement of the body.

Kinetic Energy Energy associated with movement.

Lactic Acid By-product of anaerobic glycolysis resulting from the incomplete breakdown of carbohydrate.

Ligament Connective tissue that attaches bone to bone to provide stability to the joints.

Maximal Oxygen Uptake ($\dot{V}O_2$max). The maximal rate at which oxygen can be consumed per minute; the power or capacity of the aerobic system.

Metabolism The sum total of the chemical changes or reactions occurring in the body.

Minerals Inorganic compounds, some of which are nutrients (i.e. vital to proper body functions).

Muscle Number of muscle fibres bound together by connective tissue.

Muscle Fibre A muscle cell.

Muscle Spindle A proprioceptor (sense organ which gives information concerning movements and positions of the body) located within special fibres called intrafusal fibres.

Myoglobin An oxygen-binding pigment which gives the muscle fibre its red colour. It acts as an oxygen store and aids in the diffusion of oxygen.

Neuromuscular Pertaining to the nervous and muscular systems.

Obesity Excessive body fat.

Overload To exercise a muscle or group of muscles against a resistance greater than that which is normally encountered.

Oxygen Debt The recovery oxygen uptake above the resting requirements used to replace the deficit incurred during exercise.

Phosphagens Compounds which yield inorganic phosphate and release energy when broken down. ATP and PC are phosphagens.

Phosphocreatine (PC) Chemical compound which is stored in the muscle and when broken down helps to manufacture ATP.

Point of Insertion That part of the muscle which moves a bone and is usually the distal attachment.

Point of Origin That part of the muscle which remains relatively fixed during a movement under normal circumstances and is usually the proximal attachment.

Power The rate of doing work. Work per unit of time; if one kilogram is raised one metre in one second, power is expressed as one kilogram-metre per second.

Prime Mover Name given to a muscle or muscles which are directly responsible for producing or controlling a specified joint action. Also call agonist.

Progressive Resistance Overloading a muscle or group of muscles by increasing the resistance as the muscles gain in strength throughout the duration of a training programme.

Proprioception The receipt of information from muscles and tendons, which provides information about body position and movement.

Protein An organic compound formed from amino-acids; a basic foodstuff – forms muscle tissue, hormones, enzymes, etc.

Pulse Rate The frequency of waves which travel down the artery after each contraction of the heart.

Repetition Maximum (RM) The maximum load a muscle or group of muscles can lift in a given number of repetitions before fatiguing. For example, a 5-RM is the maximum load which can be lifted five times.

Respiration The uptake of oxygen from the atmosphere into the lungs and then via the blood to the tissues, and exhale of carbon dioxide from the tissues to the atmosphere.

Skinfold A pinch of skin and subcutaneous fat from which total body fat can be estimated.

Supra-Sternal Notch Notch of bone at the upper end of the sternum. It can be located at the base of the neck on either side

Tendon Connective tissue often cord-like in appearance which connects muscles to bones and other structures.

Vitamin Organic nutrient in the presence of which metabolic reactions occur.

Index